FOREVER FIT *and* FABULOUS:

A Guide to Health and Vigor —Even at 70 and Beyond

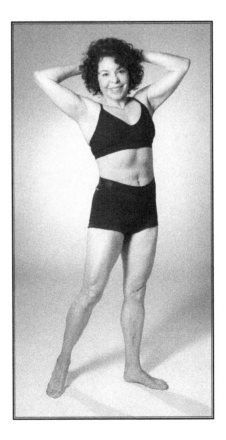

EMELINA EDWARDS

FOREVER FIT and FABULOUS:

A Guide to Health and Vigor
—Even at 70 and Beyond

by

EMELINA EDWARDS

SOUL GARDEN PRESS

MALDEN-ON-HUDSON, NEW YORK

Edwards, Emelina
Forever Fit and Fabulous,
A Guide to Health and Vigor—Even at 70 and Beyond
ISBN: 978-0-615-58126-2
1. Health and Fitness 2. Weight Training 3. Vital Aging

DISCLAIMERS

1. This book is written as a source of information only. This information is not to be considered a substitute for the advice of a qualified medical professional. Please be sure to consult your doctor before starting this or any other nutritional or exercise regimen. All the exercises in this book should be carefully studied and clearly understood before attempting them at home. The author and the publisher expressly disclaim responsibility for any adverse effects, damages, or losses arising from the use or application of the information contained therein.

2. Names and some characteristics of individuals portrayed in this book have been changed to completely protect the confidentiality of each.

To my sons, Daniel and Jacques: You are my inspiration for living the fit life.

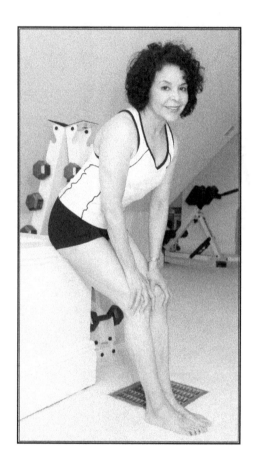

...and to All the Women

I *also dedicate this book to all the women—over the last 25 years—who have supported and inspired me.*

One of you inspired me to write my very first article some 20 years ago. Aghast when I asked you to do 20 reps of a leg exercise, you responded saying, "That's fine for you to say, how old are you anyway, 24?" I replied laughing, "That's my youngest son's age. I'm 51."

"You're kidding!" you said, excitedly curling up to face me, "Tell me everything, tell me what you eat, how much exercise you do, tell me everything!"

Your response planted the seed that sparked my courage to write when I didn't believe I could, knowing how when I had spoken to groups that I shook with fright.

Just recently one of you emailed me the most touching message I've ever received about my work: "Your life 25 years ago," you wrote, "is my life of today. I'm divorced, depressed, have no job and I can't stand that I'm so fat. But I want to be the Emelina Edwards of my generation."

I want you to know that you can be. That's one of the reasons I wrote this book.

"I feel that I am on a journey and that God is leading me to the right people and places that I need to be in order to keep me on track to fulfill my life's purpose," another one of you wrote. "I look forward to the publication of your book."

We have been there for each other, as you can see. I have drawn as much from you as you have from me. Together, we have been traveling the same road, looking for health, happiness, peace and wellness. You could even say we have written this book of change and transformation together.

When I began writing this book, I didn't intend for it to be so personal, but after all, what are we here for, if not to touch each other's hearts?

Acknowledgments

In the creation of this book I have many people to thank, but especially my patient and encouraging editor, Catharine Clarke of Soul Garden Press, along with photographer Donna Matherne of Face-to-Face Photography.

I also wish to thank the ten clients featured in Chapter 8, "The Forever Fit and Fabulous Generation," who patiently allowed me to photograph them and who shared their testimonials. I am forever grateful.

And to all others, who throughout my 25-year career, sought my advice and followed my teachings, my wish is for you to be well and happy.

God bless.

Emelina Edwards
New Orleans, Louisiana
December, 2011

❧

Contents

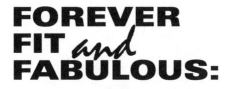

A Guide to Health and Vigor
—Even at 70 and Beyond

ॐ

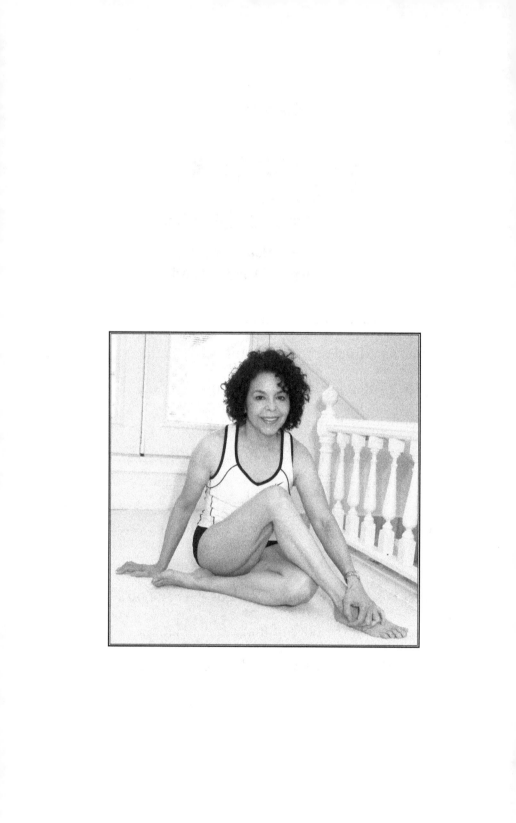

How do you see yourself in 10, 20 or 30 years? Will you be healthy, fit and fabulous, with enough vigor to do all of the things you've always dreamed of doing? Will you be happy with yourself and treasure your body? Will you be living life with courage and passion? Will your pain-free body and zest for life be a source of inspiration to your loved ones?

If you answered "yes" to all of the above questions, congratulations! You have found the keys to aging with vitality and zest, and your life reflects it.

But, if you shook your head "no" to some or most of the questions, this book is for you. Through its motivation and essential, proven practices, *Forever Fit and Fabulous: A Guide to Health and Vigor—Even at 70 and Beyond* will calm your fears of aging poorly. When you make the commitment to your fitness, to caring for yourself and your future, you will no longer be afraid. You will no longer fear finding yourself in the not too distant future functionally infirmed, with rickety legs and torsos, unable to breathe in the beauty of life, eventually confined to a walker or wheelchair. You can forget that grim scenario. You can welcome your 60s, 70s, 80s and even your 90s with a body stronger and a mind sharper than ever before. Join me on a journey of discovery to a world where rejuvenation is possible at any age because you will have found the keys to health and vitality.

Aging with strength and energy is not only possible, it can be glorious! Imagine yourself at 70, with a better body than you had at 40. Biologically, you can be 10, 20 or even 30 years younger than your chronological age. You can develop the strength and stamina of an athlete. You can look in the mirror with satisfaction, gratitude and confidence, as you see your reflection of beauty and personal accomplishment.

Forever Fit and Fabulous will teach you to welcome change. Inviting yourself to evolve is essential to maintaining a body and mind that operates at full capacity. Each new day is a precious gift that offers you an opportunity to transform any aspect of yourself that's holding you back or to simply improve on the previous day. As you well know, when you stop evolving, your body (and mind) slip into decay—and none of us want that.

Sometimes you meet someone at just the right moment who sheds light on a lingering issue or sparks a totally new way of thinking that you hadn't considered before. Or, you might read a passage that prompts an Ah-ha! moment and a ray of light brightens a dark spot.

Perhaps that's why you picked up this book. The words "forever fit and fabulous" may have attracted you. After years of putting off getting in shape, now you are ready! You're tired of feeling guilty for neglecting yourself. Or, maybe you're thinking that this book might help you recommit to the last promise you made to yourself to get fit once and for all. Now you're ten years older and feeling worse than ever, expecting more physical decline as the years go by. But help is here. Trust that *Forever Fit and Fabulous* can guide you to create your new world of vibrant, optimum health—with the pain-free body of your dreams and the fearless mentally of a yogi.

First I want to share my own story with you. The fantastic world of optimum health of body, mind and spirit has not always been mine. I created my new world after my old one fell apart.

Nearly 25 years ago, I was sickly and depressed, feeling

powerless to change my dysfunctional life. Too long stuck and miserable had taken a toll on my health. I had suffered through a cancer diagnosis, was told twice I was going blind and had a spinal deterioration that would eventually need surgery. Making matters even worse, I ended up divorced and broke. I was only 46 years old.

All this may sound like more than anyone could bear, but, for me, these multiple misfortunes lit a fire whose flame still burns. The passion of this fire inspired and motivated me to take full charge of my destiny and to create the life I had always wanted but didn't believe I could—or deserved—to have.

Intuitively I knew that to create this new life, I needed both a new mindset and a rejuvenated body. A new mindset would help me make sense of my broken life so I could free myself from unresolved issues and emotional turmoil. So I set out to study psychology. I wanted to know why I had acted destructively and how I could change my limiting habits into productive ones. My second goal—a healthier body—would give me the strength, stamina and confidence to face whatever challenges came my way with courage to grow from each experience.

Throughout this journey I learned from many teachers, but I will mention the three who influenced me the most:

✓ **Rachel McLish**[1], Ms. Olympia of 1980 and 1982, author of *Flex Appeal,* showed me that a strong, muscular body could be beautiful at a time when women considered muscles unsightly and gyms the domain of sweaty male bodies.

✓ **Drs. William Evans** and **Irwin H. Rosenberg** [2], authors

---

[1]   McLish, Rachel, *Flex Appeal* (New York: Grand Central Publishing, 1984)
[2]   Evans, William, Ph. D. and Rosenberg , Irwin H., M.D. with Thompson, Jacqueline, *Biomarkers: The 10 Determinants of Aging You Can Control* (New York: Simon & Schuster, 1991)

of *Biomarkers: The 10 Determinants of Aging You Can Control,* taught me that the aging process can be reversed and slowed down no matter what your age. The doctors were researchers on the physiology of aging, sports performance and nutrition at Tufts University when they wrote *Biomarkers.*

✓ **Dr. Deepak Chopra**[3], leading expert on mind/body medicine and author of *Ageless Body, Timeless Mind – The Quantum Alternative To Growing Old* taught me that the body is at the service of the mind and that how we think about ourselves and the world not only effects our health but also determines how slowly or quickly we age.

I began my quest for health with daily exercise, lifting weights and jogging. I lowered my intake of sugar and fat, and gave up alcohol. Within only a few months I began to feel and look better. In less than eight months I dropped two dress sizes and, for the first time in my life, had strength and energy. My depression lifted and my back strengthened, so I could straighten up instead of walking like an old lady. Amazed and excited by the impressive results I'd achieved in such a short time, I asked myself the question: Why isn't everyone doing this?

The answer came: Start teaching!

For the next 25 years I taught, wrote fitness articles, made TV and radio appearances and presented my innovative fitness program to business groups and conventioneers. I produced a home workout video, a cookbook and a relaxation tape. Wanting to also reach Latino audiences, I flew to Miami and on the "Cristina Show" on the Spanish network Univision urged

---

[3] Chopra, Deepak *Ageless Body, Timeless Mind – The Quantum Alternative To Growing Old* (New York: Harmony Books, 1993)

Latinos to empower themselves by strengthening their bodies, which would have a positive ripple effect on their minds and their souls. When The Home Shopping Network en Español came calling, I went on the show, waking up sleepyheads at 7AM with my health and fitness message.

As passionate as I was then about my message, I am even more enthusiastic now, for I have not been sick in bed once in the last two decades! I train everyday with gusto for what it gives me, and for what it gives my two sons—a healthy, strong, happy and resourceful mother. I believe that my greatest legacy will be the example I have set for them and for my grandchildren. When Sophie, my first grandchild, celebrated her very first birthday, I gave her a miniature workout bench and weights! Growing up in a home of athletes, she couldn't help but be inspired. At age eight, she realized her first dream, a junior black belt in Taekwondo.

When I thought about writing this book, I immediately knew what the title would be: *Forever Fit and Fabulous: A Guide to Health and Vigor—Even at 70 and Beyond.* Yes, you can erase almost half of your age by how you live your life. I call this "radical aging". This book offers you radical ideas to slow, and, in many cases, reverse the passage of time. I'm not referring to the latest anti-aging cream or youth hormone, but time-proven, safe and practical methods to prevent and often reverse the ravages of time. You already possess everything you need to live life to the fullest with optimum health, vigor and vitality for the rest of your life.

Join me as we discover the marvel of your body and find new ways to take care of your most precious asset. As inspiration I offer you both my personal experience and the scientific information that gave me back my life. Read on and begin to realize your dreams.

❧

CHAPTER ONE:
Muscles, Your Power Source

*"Muscle mass and strength can be regained, no matter what
your age and no matter what the state of your body's musculature
before you start your exercise program."*

—William Evans, Ph. D. and Irwin H. Rosenberg, M. D.[1]

(Authors of *Biomarkers: The 10 Determinants of Aging You Can Control.*

Dr. William Evans is professor of Geriatrics at Duke University and Dr. Rosenberg
is Doctor of Internal Medicine in Boson, Massachusetts.)

If my Introduction has inspired you to begin working out
right away, leave this chapter for later reading and go directly
to Chapter 5, my Vibrant Health Workout program. There's not
a minute to waste! Start pumping, sweating and breathing your
way into the best shape of your life. But, if you need a bit more
information and encouragement to get you going, keep reading.

In 1991, after working out for four years and witnessing the
phenomenal transformation of my own middle-aged body, as
mentioned in the Introduction, I read a recently published book

---

[1] Evans, Williams, Ph.D. and Rosenberg, Irwin H., M.D. with Thompson,
Jacqueline, Biomarkers: The 10 Determinants of Aging You Can Control (New
York: Simon & Schuster, 1991)

called *Biomarkers: The 10 Determinants of Aging You Can Control.*[2] Written by William Evans, Ph.D. and Irwin H. Rosenberg, M. D., the book describes the results of their landmark study at the USDA Human Nutrition Center on Aging at Tufts University.

Evans and Rosenberg had put male senior citizens aged 60 to 70 through a 12-week program of weight training. After only 12 weeks, their strength had increased by almost 200%! [3] Their muscles got both bigger and stronger. The women in the study ranged in ages from 87 to 96, and they also showed remarkable results. Their strength levels tripled and they increased their muscle size by 10%! These impressive results proved that, contrary to popular opinion, muscle loss is completely preventable and reversible at any age, even 90.

Regardless of your body's physical condition when you begin, you can still make gains. The principal message of the *Biomarkers* study reveals: many physiological declines of aging can be reversed, or at the very least improved.

When we choose not to take action to improve our health, our bodies' deterioration as we age is as dramatic—in the opposite direction—as the results of the Tufts study. In our mid-20s we begin to lose muscle mass. In our 30s we begin to lose strength and stamina, and start gaining weight. In our 40s, the rate of muscle loss accelerates, shifting our body composition to fat over muscle. Over 50 and into our 60s, we have lost most of our strength and stamina and we've slowed down.

By our 70s many of us begin to consider what assisted living program we'll be able to afford, because we have come to believe that the deterioration of our bodies is inevitable and that chronic

---

[2] Ibid. p. 7
[3] Ibid. p. 14

conditions like heart disease, diabetes, cancer and fractures are a part of aging. Weak and decrepit, many of us will spend the rest of our lives complaining of ailments and comparing doctors.

The muscle loss and brittle bones that come as the result of not improving our health now set the stage for serious illnesses like osteoporosis. Life now becomes painful and difficult. We begin to move stiffly and to suffer chronic aches and pains.

But it's never too late to postpone disability and reduce your risk for chronic diseases. You can regain your muscular strength by developing muscle mass, the vital ingredient for the support of your entire body. As you "work" your muscles and other parts of your body, you can also learn to take care of your body, to appreciate and love it for what it does for you.

Imagine my surprise when I read *Biomarkers* and realized that while I had been training and teaching clients in my own little corner of the world, Tufts scientists Evans and Rosenberg had also been training people with results that scientifically proved what I knew intuitively: middle-aged spread has nothing to do with age, but rather with body composition. And who is responsible for the body composition lean toward fat over muscle? We are! It's our sedentary lifestyle that perpetuates our accumulated fat and loss of muscle.

I thought back on my poor eating habits of the past, stuffing myself with cheese, butter, cream, all kinds of meats, rich sauces and alcoholic drinks—all of which caused by body fat to skyrocket. Meanwhile, my stressful, sedentary living had eaten away my muscle mass. My body was in such shock that my digestive system wasn't working properly; I suffered from chronic constipation. Even though I was only slightly overweight, by about 20 pounds, I was obese due to my body composition.

3

In addition to my dangerous body composition, my disuse and misuse of my body lead to a "deteriorating spine" diagnosis that I was told would eventually need surgery.

Gratefully, due to my weight training program and improved diet, I left that threat in the past. After reading *Biomarkers*, I knew for certain that as long as I lived I would never again neglect my body. Getting to know my body through the process of restoring my health day in and day out has given me a new appreciation for my body. I now welcome the daily challenge of building strength, stamina and flexibility. My mantra became: *Learn to love what's good for you!*

The road to knowing, appreciating and loving my body has been long and hard. I still remember how I used to blame my body and want to punish it whenever I suffered a symptom. With a mind totally disconnected from my body, I treated it as a separate entity.

One particular incident comes to mind. I awoke one morning with red bumps all over my face and arms. Alarmed and scared, I hurried to see a dermatologist. Nothing like that had ever happened to me before. The doctor looked at my face, wrote a prescription and told me to apply the cream until the red bumps disappeared.

Every day I scrubbed the cream on my face and arms as hard as I could, as if to punish my skin for daring to displease me. A few weeks later I noticed that instead of red bumps, I now had white patches all over my face and arms. Again in a panic, I returned to the dermatologist and showed him the white patches. He looked at me with a calm and casual manner and said, "Oh, that's just the side effect of the drug."

Furious at the doctor for not warning me that the cure could be worse than the symptom, I vowed to scratch him off my list.

As for my ailing body, I still had not learned empathy for myself. I didn't realize that the stress caused by my chaotic life had also caused my skin to break-out. The rash on my face and arms was my body's message to look inward and make changes to restore her to balance and health.

Have you had a similar experience? What do you do when a symptom stops you dead in your tracks? Do you blame your body and want to punish it as I once did or are you kinder to yourself?

When you understand that the mind impacts the body and symptoms originate in the mind, you'll know where to look for a solution. Your body will ask (or demand) that you change an attitude, a habit or a behavior that has created the symptom.

As the chapters in this book unfold, you'll see how building strength, stamina and flexibility will awaken within you a deeper appreciation and love for your body and you too will intend to never neglect it again.

10 DETERMINANTS OF AGING YOU CAN CONTROL

The 10 Determinants of Aging You Can Control reveal how your daily choices control how your body ages, and what you can do to slow and reverse its inevitable functional decline. You are not a victim of your aging body; rather, your aging body responds to your decisions.

The ten physical aspects of aging or "biomarkers" that you can control through lifestyle changes are: your muscle mass, your strength, your basal metabolic rate, your body fat percentage, your aerobic capacity, your blood pressure, your insulin sensitivity, your cholesterol HDL ratio, your bone density and your body temperature regulation.[4]

---

[4] Ibid, p. 42

Your muscle mass.[5] Scientific studies have shown that we begin to lose muscle mass in our mid-20s at the rate of 6.6 pounds every ten years. That's roughly one half pound per year. This rate accelerates as we enter our 40s.

Several of my 70-something clients have come to me with complaints about struggling to get out of the car or the bathtub. I immediately have them focus on their leg workout and start them on squats if they are not already doing them. I believe it is essential to develop strong leg muscles and a strong hip area by working the muscles used when bending at the knee. Each of my clients eventually learns how to do squats, the king of exercises that strengthen legs and hip areas. Squat mimics the act of sitting, getting up from a sitting position, and then going down again. Every time we squat, we fortify the joints, muscles, nerves and ligaments in the leg and hip area.

If you cannot squat due to knee, ankle or hip problems, you can do Donkey Kicks (see page 85), an alternative exercise that strengthens the same muscles as the squat.

Your strength.[6] is totally dependent on your muscle mass. If you increase muscle mass, you increase strength.

Muscle plays such a huge role in reversing and retarding the aging process because building and maintaining muscle tissue affects not only the "strength" biomarker, but also all the other biomarkers as well.

After my first son Daniel was born, I had 20 pounds of extra weight that I could not lose. I decided running could be my last hope. So I went to the track and started to run, but my legs wouldn't do what I wanted them to. They felt like lead. Unable to breathe properly, I gasped for air and a painful cramp caught

[5] Ibid, p. 44
[6] Ibid, p. 46

in my side. Feeling frustrated and defeated, I swore never to run again because it was not for me. Fast forward 46 years—today, at age 70, after 25 years of training, with strong muscles, fit lungs and a well-hydrated body, I can run without difficulty.

Conditioning made the difference between these two scenarios. My body, at 70, is better prepared for any challenge, than it was when I was in my 20s.

Have you ever had a similar experience? Did you at one time attempt an activity but when unsuccessful gave up, angry and disappointed at your failure?

If so, you too can revisit and triumph over a past experience that left you dissatisfied. It's never too late to prove to yourself that you can do it. Conditioning your body is key. You too can build strength, stamina, breathe deeply and hydrate your body, preparing it for any activity you wish to undertake. For more inspiration, read the stories in Chapter 8, "The Forever Fit and Fabulous Generation".

*Your **BMR, or basal metabolic rate*** [7] measures the rate at which your body burns energy at low exertion. The more muscle you have, the more calories you burn. The less muscle you have, the fewer calories your body will burn.

Beginning at age 20, BMR drops two percent per decade. By the time you're 50, your BMI has dropped by eight percent and reduces your body's ability to burn the calories from your food intake. Unless you stop this decline by taking up weight training to increase your lean muscle mass, *your body will continue to accumulate more and more fat.*

After I graduated high school I weighed 140 pounds. I couldn't stand myself and wanted desperately to lose the 25 pounds that I

---

[7] Ibid, p. 52

had gained. When I told a friend of my misery, she handed me a cigarette and told me that smoking would keep my hunger away. So, I started to smoke. For weeks I lived on cigarettes and coffee and lost ten pounds. One day I woke up on my bedroom floor without any memory of how I had gotten there. My malnourished body had gone into shock and overdosed during the night on cold medicine. If I had been eating a healthy diet and not smoking, my body could have withstood the extra dose of medicine.

Women of all ages complain that their bulging waistlines create their greatest source of dissatisfaction with their bodies. Starvation diets or smoking offer no solution and can be extremely dangerous. Eating a nutritious diet (see Chapter 6, Nutrition: You Are What You Eat) and increasing your metabolism (see Chapter 5, the Vibrant Health Workout) allow you to burn calories even at rest.

Your body fat percentage.[8] Unless you train like an athlete, getting older means gaining body fat. Even if your body looks relatively the same and you haven't gained much weight, chances are that your lean body mass has decreased and your fat increased. Evans and Rosenberg have estimated that the average sedentary 65-year-old female consists of about 43% fat. This bears repeating. *The average sedentary 65-year-old female is about 43% fat.*[9]

Do you know your BMI? Your Body Mass Index calculates your weight in relation to height. This figure assesses your risk for developing the chronic diseases associated with aging. It also helps you determine your risk for dying prematurely and shows

[8] Ibid, p. 53
[9] Ibid, p. 53

you how much weight you must lose to prevent all of the above. To find out your BMI, Google BMI, and on the BMI calculator page, fill in two blanks, one for height and the other for weight. You will get an instant BMI reading. Compare your BMI to ideal ratings for your age, also found on the same page. If your BMI is 20 percent or more above ideal values, you are obese, and your weight problem can place you at risk of dying younger than necessary.

I know how tough it can be to face this truth, but we cannot change what we don't acknowledge. If you want to feel better, look better and have more energy than ever before, you must know where you stand. Then you can begin to look forward to the dramatic changes you can create in the years to come, as my client Carolyn did.

Carolyn shares her story in Chapter 8, The Forever Fit and Fabulous Generation. She lowered her BMI from 37 to 29 by losing 45 pounds—now close to ideal for her age. Carolyn is no longer at risk for heart disease, diabetes or cancer. To reverse her high-fat/low-muscle ratio, Carolyn began lifting weights and changed her diet to include more high-fiber, low-fat and low-sugar foods. Her added muscle has helped her speed her metabolism and her improved diet has helped her burn fat.

Aerobic capacity [10] implies the capacity to bring oxygen into the lungs and deliver blood to the heart where the bloodstream can effectively pump blood to all parts of the body.

If you have led a sedentary life, as I did until I was 46 years old, your aerobic capacity has declined. If you're 65, it's been reduced by 30 to 40 percent! Your heart cannot function to full capacity if you're aerobically unfit. Your heart needs strong, healthy lungs

---

[10] Ibid, p. 60

to process oxygen throughout your whole body.

When I started jogging at 46, my aerobic capacity had been severely compromised. At first I could barely jog a few yards before I had to stop to give my chest a rest. I then walked a few paces and a few minutes later picked up the pace again. I continued walking and jogging until my lungs got used to the new level of exertion. I struggled for weeks, but eventually I was able to double and then triple the distance, until I could finally jog a whole mile.

Dr. Kenneth H. Cooper (the father of aerobics) says that for minimal aerobic benefit, 20 to 30 minutes of aerobic activity (walking, jogging, cycling), three to four times per week is sufficient. He also recommends that the aerobic activity be performed continuously, uninterrupted, rather than breaking it up into segments throughout the day.

Be patient with yourself, but start walking, jogging, climbing stairs, riding a bike, jumping rope or whatever suits you—the key is to do it! Don't wait until barely a wisp of air travels through your lungs, hampering blood flow to the rest of your body. Give your heart and lungs the aerobic activity they need.

Your body's ability to process blood sugar [11] is, like most of the other biomarkers, negatively affected by your elevated fat level and reduced muscle mass. Elevated blood sugar levels increase the risk of developing Type 2 Diabetes and in turn raise the risk of heart disease. After age 70, 20 percent of men and 30 percent of women become at risk for developing diabetes.

I grew up eating a very unhealthy diet: fried meats and fowl, vegetables cooked in lard and fruits soaked in sugar. Fat or sugar or both coated everything I remember eating. As an adult, I

---

[11] Ibid, p. 67

continued to eat the same way I had as a child, unaware that my diet could eventually kill me.

And it almost did. A combination of poor diet, chronic stress and anxiety, psychic suffering and sedentary living no doubt caused the cancer I contracted in my early 40s. My decision to get fit and change my diet put a halt to my deteriorating health. If I hadn't made these changes, I would now be among the millions of Latinas suffering from diabetes.

According to The Federal Office of Minority Health[12], 73 percent of Mexican-American women are overweight or obese, as compared to 61 percent of the general female population. Hispanic children have a 1:2 (one in two) chance of developing diabetes in their lifetime, as compared to 1:3 (one in three) for the general population.

A prevention campaign developed by the National Diabetes Education Program and the National Institutes of Health and the Centers for Disease Control and Prevention[13] highlights some good news: by losing a small amount of weight, limiting fat and caloric intake and exercising 30 minutes a day, 5 days a week, the risk for diabetes can be reduced by *more than half!*

Your cholesterol ratio.[14] Our body produces some cholesterol naturally (blood cholesterol) and other cholesterol comes from the foods we eat (dietary cholesterol). High amounts of cholesterol in the blood can create cholesterol deposits in the bloodstream known as atherosclerosis that contributes to the development of heart disease.

When I changed my diet from animal-based to plant-based, I drastically reduced my cholesterol level. Cholesterol is found only

---

12 http://minorityhealth.hhs.gov/templates/content.aspx?lvl=3&lvlID=537&ID=6459
13 http://www.nih.gov/news/pr/jun2004/niddk-29.htm
14 Ibid, p. 71

in animal-based foods. Today the only animal-based food I eat is an occasional serving of fish or egg or a tiny piece of cheese.

If your cholesterol level is dangerously high, consider reducing your intake of animal-based foods. Eat more fruits, vegetables, whole grains, beans, seeds and nuts. For more information on a plant-based diet, see Chapter 6, complete with recipes.

Your blood pressure.[15] Abnormally high blood pressure called "hypertension" has multiple causes: genetic predisposition, obesity, a salty diet, excessive alcohol consumption, smoking and a sedentary lifestyle. Hypertension is a risk factor for heart disease and stroke.

I have a genetic predisposition for hypertension, but I control it through exercise, meditation and diet. I exercise every day and meditate twice daily. It's amazing to experience how meditation can lower heartbeat, pulse and respiration. The body actually rests in space, completely still, in perfect balance.

If you suffer from hypertension, you must eat healthy, exercise vigorously and meditate on a regular basis—always considering your doctor's advice. For tips on meditation, see Chapter 7.

Your bone density.[16] Over the course of a lifetime, the average woman's thighbone that joins with the hip decreases by 55 percent—a primary reason that older women fall and break bones.[17]

Whenever I see someone walking hunched over it reminds me of my old self. If I had not started lifting weights when I did, I would now be crippled with osteoporosis. My spine, already deteriorating in my early 30s, would not have been able to support my upper body.

[15] Ibid, p. 75
[16] Ibid, p. 77
[17] Ibid, p. 78

Osteoporosis is not a normal consequence of aging. It's a preventable disease. When you weight train, you exert pressure on your bones and make them stronger. Other weight-bearing exercises that prevent bone loss are walking, running and cycling.

Regardless of your age, you can prevent osteoporosis, broken bones and nursing homes—by getting serious about lifting weights to strengthen your bones and the muscles designed to protect them.

Regulating your internal temperature.[18] Your body's ability to regulate its own internal temperature diminishes with age. If you are aerobically unfit and sedentary, you may have lost the ability to sweat. When we don't sweat, blood flow to the skin diminishes. Heat build-up in the body would normally escape as sweat. With heat trapped inside the body internal temperatures can soar to dangerous levels.

Before I changed my lifestyle, I was always hot. I could not stand the heat and humidity in New Orleans. I complained constantly and dreaded summers. Today, summer is my favorite time of the year. I can walk comfortably in 90-degree weather and hardly need air conditioning. My lifestyle made the difference. Today I drink plenty of water and sweat every day. My meditation practice also lowers my body temperature.

By drinking lots of water, engaging in regular exercise and also meditating, you too can increase your body's ability to release heat through sweat and maintain a lower body temperature. Exercise, drink water and meditate to enjoy a cool body.

So there you have them—the ten key physiological factors associated with aging *that are, each and every one of them, under your control!* As you can see, muscle and strength are at the top of

---

[18] Ibid, p. 81

the list, because when these diminish, your over all functioning will be at risk. You will then lose your independence and your ability to move at will. Beyond that point, life as you know it will never be the same.

When I read *Biomarkers* soon after its publication 20 years ago, I felt truly blessed. Elated, I wanted to fly to Boston and personally thank the two men who had scientifically proven the basis of my lifework: lifting weights as essential to fitness, health and longevity. Or, as I would say to my clients: build muscle or get fat, weak and frail!

Biomarkers affirmed and acknowledged my intuition and faith that restoring muscle restores health. During my early years of personal training, naysayers considered weight lifting a passing fad. When I shared what I did with others, some laughed, saying "And people actually *pay* you to train them?" or "You make a living doing *that?*"

Biomarkers removed those doubts and offered scientific proof to the naysayers. With *Biomarkers* as support for my gut feelings, my career carried new meaning as an avid advocate of weight lifting. I knew from experience that weight lifting could change lives but now I had the expertise of renowned scientists at a prestigious institution substantiating what I had known all along.

With the publication of *Biomarkers*, the value of weight training shifted from recreational to medical. Up until the early 90s, only bodybuilders pumped iron, training their muscles for size and definition and competing for titles and prizes. But the good work of Tufts University scientists, William Evans, Ph. D. and Irwin H. Rosenberg, M. D. gave building muscle an essential new purpose: preserving muscle function and vitality and staying young longer.

In 1998, some seven years after the publication of *Biomarkers*, Dr. Kenneth H. Cooper, founder of the Cooper Aerobic Center in Dallas, Texas, published *Regaining the Power of Youth at Any Age* [19]. His book concludes that after his evaluation of scientific data and his own experience with aerobic and strength training over more than 30 years, that the percentage of aerobic work versus weight work needs to be adjusted by different age groups. For example, 51 to 60 year-olds need 60 percent aerobic work and 40 percent strength; 61 and older (my category) need 55 percent aerobic and 45 percent strength. This adjustment reflects his current belief that aerobic and muscle needs vary with age.

Dr. Cooper emphasizes that both aerobic and strength training are essential to slow down the physical deterioration of aging and to regain some of the energy and youthfulness of our younger years.

So what kinds of gains can you expect to make once you begin your exercise program?

Dr. Cooper cites a 1989 report (*Journal of Applied Physiology*, Vol. 66, No. 6, pp. 2589-94) on a study by University of Florida researchers. A group of 70 to 79 healthy, untrained men and women were split into three groups: one group performed aerobic type exercises (cycling, treadmill-walking), another group did resistance (weight lifting) work and the third group did nothing. Their physical training consisted of three sessions per week for 26 weeks.

At the end of the study, the aerobic training group increased their oxygen uptake by 22 percent, and the resistance-training group increased their lower body strength by 9 percent and their

---

[19] Cooper, Kenneth H., Dr., *Regaining the Power of Youth at Any Age*, (Nashville: Thomas Nelson Publishing, 2005)

upper body strength by 18 percent.

The researchers concluded that healthy men and women in their 70s can reap positive benefits by engaging in prolonged and challenging exercise training. And, says Dr. Cooper, what the study proved to him is that if older people are willing to train, they can *regain the power of youth!*

In 2010, Dr. Walter M. Bortz, II, eminent gerontologist, passionate promoter of exercise and a lifelong marathoner—he ran his 40th marathon at 80—published *The Roadmap to 100.*[20] He believes that inactivity is the single leading cause of health issues. He cites several studies, each more compelling than the other, that prove time and again that to live a life worth living, exercise is key.

In his book, Dr. Bortz cites a particular longitudinal study by a team of Harvard researchers.[21] The participants were several thousand 70-year-old men who were in basic good health. The scientists hoped to find the key to a healthy long life aside from genetics. The study showed that regular exercise resulted in a nearly 30 percent lower mortality risk and that those who lived a healthy lifestyle (did not smoke, were not diabetic, obese or hypertensive and exercised) had a 54 percent chance of living to 90 or beyond. In addition, they enjoyed better physical function, mental well-being and lower incidence of the chronic diseases associated with aging.

Dr. Bortz emphasizes that lifestyle, not genetics is the key to longevity.

---

[20] Bortz II, Walter M. M.D. and Stickrod, Randall *The Roadmap to 100: The Breakthrough Science of Living A Long and Healthy Life* (New York: Palgrave Macmillian, 2010) p. 31, 33, 41

[21] Ibid, p. 71

In discussing the impact of lifestyle on health, such a discussion is incomplete without emphasizing the impact of physical neglect on our brains and its functioning.

The Alzheimer's Association describes Alzheimer's as a progressive and fatal brain disease. As many as 5.3 million Americans are living with Alzheimer's, and some 500,000 people in their 30s, 40s, and 50s have Alzheimer's disease or a related dementia.

In *The Roadmap to 100*, Dr. Bortz quotes Dr. Ronald Petersen, director of the Alzheimer's Research Center at the Mayo Clinic: "Regular physical exercise is probably the best means we have of preventing Alzheimer's disease today, better than medications, better than intellectual activity, better than supplements and diet."

Dr. Bortz also points out that Columbia University Medical Center found in physically active volunteers that the risk of Alzheimer's decreased by a third. Those who combined exercise with a healthy diet high in fruits and vegetables lowered their risk by 60 percent! He adds that these recent findings have received little public attention because perhaps most of that attention focuses on pharmaceutical efforts.

Short-term memory loss is one the most common signs of Alzheimer's and typically can disrupt daily life. We've all heard that to keep our brainpower from deteriorating we must regularly challenge, train and use our brains just as we should our bodies if we want to remain vital and energetic. Through lack of use, our brains can atrophy, blocking and breaking down the connections that aid in memory. Fortunately, there are several things we can do to prevent such devastation—for one, we can exercise!

Exercise can strengthen nerve cells by increasing blood and energy supply to the brain. This stimulates the release of growth factors and BDNF, a substance that promotes branching of neurons, inducing nerve cells to grow, branch and make connections with one another and, in some cases, produce new nerve cells.

In his book entitled *Spark*, John J. Ratey, M. D., clinical associate professor of psychiatry at Harvard Medical School, and also author of *The User's Guide to the Brain*, states that the central message of *Spark* is to convince the reader to exercise, because exercise is *the single most powerful tool available to improve brain function.* Dr. Ratey bases this statement on evidence he has gathered from hundreds of recent research papers. He notes that not only neuroscientists, but also kinesiologists and epidemiologists, concur that the more fit we are, the better our brain works. Ratey goes on to say: "The research consistently shows that the more fit you are, the more resilient your brain becomes, and the better it functions cognitively and psychologically. If you get your body in shape, your mind will follow."

As you can see, the science in favor of exercise is overwhelming. The choice is now up to you. How you choose to live your life, caring for or ignoring your health, will determine how you will function in your later years. Your choices now will impact your body for the rest of your life. Give your body the extra muscle it needs to support your longevity. Make a promise to yourself to begin now! Don't waste another day!

ভৈ

CHAPTER TWO
Reprogramming Outdated Beliefs

"Your subconscious mind is working right now, day and night, to make sure that you become precisely the person you have unconsciously described yourself to be." [1]

—Shad Helmstetter, Ph. D.

(Shad Helmstetter Ph. D., is a leading behavioral psychologist and authority in the field of Self-Management. He is the author of What to Say When You Talk to Yourself *and* Winning From Within.*)*

Your body is a product of your beliefs. Throughout your entire life, your thoughts, words, feelings and emotions have influenced your decisions and actions.

Such decisions may seem insignificant but have a major impact. Let's begin with your morning snack. Did you choose the doughnut or the apple? After work, did you put on your walking shoes and hit the park or curl up on the couch with a bowl of ice cream? Have you given up on yourself because you have lost faith in your ability to lose weight or do you keep challenging yourself to reach your weight goals? When you realize you are gaining

---

[1] Helmstetter, Shad Ph. D. *What To Say When You Talk To Yourself* (New York: MJF Books, 1986)

weight, do you get back on track with your exercise program promising yourself *this* time it will be different or do you just buy a larger dress size?

Each moment-by-moment decision across the course of your life has led to how you look and feel today, healthy and strong, weak and sickly or somewhere in between.

Every thought you think—conscious or unconscious—directs the control centers in your brain to electrically and chemically affect your every feeling and action. All of your thoughts have the power to program your mind and body and to direct your life.

Until I started lifting weights, the body I had created was not the one I wanted. In magazines and books I saw photos of women with strong and beautiful bodies, but didn't believe I was rich enough, young enough or lucky enough to look like one of them. I did not believe in the power of effort and dedication. I did not believe that desire and hard work could motivate me to accomplish anything. Also, I was strongly influenced by cultural conditioning that said, "If the women in your family look like this, this is how you will also look, and there's nothing you can do about it."

When I looked into the mirror, I thought my only option was resigning myself to my genetic fate. Looking for solutions to change my body didn't even enter my consciousness.

In light of my mental state at that time, it's no wonder I was not ready to make the connection between my actions and their consequences. I continued my unhealthy living habits until my rash of illnesses—cancer, near blindness, and degenerative disease of the cervical spine—unbearably escalated and woke me up to a new reality. I realized that I had to make different choices in order to create healthier outcomes. I could no longer blame genetics, my age, my bank account, or the weather. Only I was responsible for my condition and only I could turn it around.

I wanted permanent change, something I could hold on to for the rest of my life, something that would help me to create and maintain the body and the life I wanted. One afternoon I was browsing in a bookstore and picked up a book called *What To Say When You Talk To Yourself* [2] by Shad Helmstetter, Ph.D. The title got my attention, and I bought it. The book changed my life.

Dr. Helmstetter's message is simple and straightforward: Your success or failure in anything, large or small, will depend on your programming—both what you accept from others and what you say when you talk to yourself. This is a simple fact, and neither luck nor desire have anything to do with it. *The brain simply believes what you most tell it. You will become what you most think about. What you put in your brain results in what comes out of it, disguised as behavior.*

Belief does not require something to be true, only that we believe it to be true. We create our realities based upon what we have come to believe, whether true or not!

I used to believe that my protruding belly, skinny legs and flat butt were the products of genetics, because I shared this body type with other women in my family. Since I couldn't fight genetics, I believed that there was nothing I could do about it. But, when I started weight training and cut back on fat and sugar, I found out that I had been wrong. My body began to change. I realized I had the power to mold my body into the shape I wanted.

Since whatever you believe about yourself will affect what you do, let's examine some of the beliefs that may be holding you

---

[2] Ibid.

back. If you can identify with any of these, it's time to reprogram your thinking.

Exercise is torture.

Actually, exercise relieves the torture you may be suffering due to unhealthy living. Exercise can relieve your painful back, your sore shoulders and your aching joints.

Since I hit 50, my body has fallen apart and there's nothing I can do about it.

As you have gotten older, you may have gained fat and lost muscle. Menopause can also be a contributing factor. You may notice the beginnings of a "spare tire" around your middle that makes it difficult to zip your pants. You may also notice that your triceps are softer and weaker than they used to be. That's why when you lift your arm to wave, the skin under your arm swings to and fro. Your hips may also have gotten wider so you now struggle to get into your pants. But you can change your body composition through regular exercise and cutting the fat and sugar from your diet. And remember, it's never too late to build muscle. Maria A. Fiatarone, M. D., specialist in geriatric medicine, proved through her studies, that participants aged 90 and beyond were able to build as much muscle size and growth as young people doing the same amount of exercise.[3]

I can't exercise because I don't have any energy.

The listless, sluggish feeling you're suffering from is the result of sedentary living. To *get* energy and to put a zip in your step, you have to move your body. Energy comes from the oxygen you take into your lungs when you engage in physical activity. When

---

[3] http://findarticles.com/p/articles/mi_m0815/is_n211_v21/ai_18995174/

your heart rate goes up, your blood starts flowing and releases endorphins (your body's natural *feel good* chemicals) throughout your bloodstream. A strong heart gives you stamina.

I just don't have the discipline to start a workout program.

You develop and nurture your self-discipline by showing up for your well-being, day in and day out. You'll realize that when you skip a day, you miss the elation that comes with exercise and you won't want to miss it. You stop skipping it. You're hooked and realize you've got all the discipline you need.

I have terrible genes. People in my family age fast.

Your genes affect only 30 percent of your aging process. Your lifestyle determines the other 70 percent!

I'm afraid that exercise may not be good for my arthritis.

Exercise is a form of physical therapy. It can prevent your symptoms from getting worse and can even relieve your existing discomfort altogether. Ask your doctor to prescribe a modified weight-lifting program for you. You'll be amazed at how much better you will feel.

I don't have time to exercise.

How many hours a day do you spend watching television? The average American sits in front of the tube four hours a day. If you do an inventory of your time and how you spend it, you could probably find one hour a day for an activity that can save your life. You wouldn't say you don't have time to brush your teeth or take a bath, would you?

Exercise is just too hard.

What can be harder than looking in the mirror every day and disliking what you see? What can be harder than knowing that you will never realize your dream of being lean because you don't think you're worth the effort? What can be harder than being chronically sick because your immune system is low-functioning? What can be harder than seeing and feeling your body deteriorate because you would rather sit on the couch?

I can't afford to exercise.

Whatever financial investment you make for regular exercise, it will come back to you tenfold through the value of vital health. Look at it this way: you will save on doctor bills and medications and you will double your earning potential because you'll live longer. That means you'll be able to work more hours, so in the end, you'll end up with more money and will have better health to be able to enjoy it. Exercise is a down payment on the future joy of having an energetic and pain-free body. Besides, all you need to get started is a set of inexpensive free weights and my workout instructions.

I don't need to exercise; I wear a size 4 dress.

Have you ever heard the term "skinny fat"? That's slang for "normal-weight obesity" a term coined by researchers to describe more than half of all normal-weight Americans—30 million strong—who have high percentages of body fat that put them at risk for obesity-related health problems. If a woman falls into this category, she is twice as likely to die from heart problems or stroke. Without healthy eating and exercise, being merely thin is not being fit. "There are some individuals who may not be fat or obese on the outside, but they're fat or obese on the inside," said Dr. Peter Vash of the Lindora Clinic. Interviewed by Lori Corbin for an ABC news segment on the subject of "skinny fat," Dr. Vash added, "Some people may look to be at normal weight, but they have this increased deep visceral fat that causes them to have higher risk for diabetes, hypertension and heart disease."

I don't lift weights because I don't want to bulk up.

Normally, women cannot bulk up like men because they don't carry enough testosterone in their bodies. The muscle-bound professional female bodybuilders you see on TV are a rarity. These women train for a living and spend countless hours in the gym lifting enormous amounts of weight. You will be training for only one hour, twice or three times per week, and that regimen combined with consistent aerobic exercise will get you just what you want—a lean, beautiful and strong body.

STAYING TRUE TO YOURSELF

I would like to delve more deeply into this belief about bulking up. "I don't want to bulk up" may cover up the *fear of being too strong*. This isn't a conscious fear. No one says, "I don't want to lift weights because I'm afraid I might get too strong." But the unconscious fear can show up in behavior.

Years ago I was training a healthy and strong young woman named Carolyn, who was more than ready to increase the weight she was using. When I pointed out to her that she could go heavier, she panicked. "I can't do that," she said. "What if I drop the weight on my head?" Suddenly all of Carolyn's common sense disappeared. I explained to her that that was not likely to happen because her first reaction would be to lower her arm, not to let go of the weight. But Carolyn remained fearful, and soon after quit training.

As I pondered the real reason for Carolyn's decision to quit, I remembered something she had said to me during our initial visit that could have had a bearing on her decision. "I want to get in shape but my boyfriend doesn't want me to bulk up," she had said. With his warning in the back of her mind, no wonder Carolyn panicked. I suspect that she was afraid of losing her boyfriend, so she sacrificed what she wanted. Carolyn did not stay true to herself.

Over the years I have come across similar scenarios. Perfectly intelligent women fear heavier weights because someone in their lives—a critical relative, a threatened boyfriend or a jealous girlfriend—discouraged them from becoming too strong. If this has been your experience, read on.

Many years ago during a radio interview with a behavioral psychologist this very topic came up. "If we want to save ourselves," I said, "Sometimes we have to leave the group and go off on our own to find our own path. You can't be intimidated by peer disapproval. You just have to go out and make new friends, ones who will not shun you for wanting to try something new, but support your new interests." My host nodded, smiling, and then asked, "Have you ever heard of the 'crabs in a bucket theory'?"

When I shook my head, she explained that "crabs in a bucket" is a metaphor that describes the tendency of members of a group to "pull down" any member who achieves success beyond the others, out of jealousy or fear of losing them. "The analogy is to a bucket of live crabs," she said. "Whenever one crab tries to escape the bucket by climbing out of it, the others reach up and pull it down. And if that crab keeps trying time and again to climb out of the bucket, eventually the others will chew off its legs! The mentality is 'if I can't have it, neither can you.'"

When we make a move to better ourselves, it takes a strong personality to stand up to criticisms and ridicule from those close to us. You can't imagine the criticisms I endured when I started building muscle and stopped eating fat and sugar. But I was not about to let anyone stand in the way of my health.

Once, at a restaurant with an old friend, I asked the waitress to tell me the ingredients of the sauce in the dish I was considering. After the waitress left, my friend turned to me and said, "I hope you're not turning into a fanatic about eating too much fat!" Fat to her was not an issue; she had just ordered fried oysters. I didn't respond to her comment, but decided that this was the last meal I could share with her. It took years of personal growth to muster the courage to answer a similar comment with a sense of humor. Today, I would simply laugh and order what I want.

So don't be the crab in the bucket! Don't get pulled down (or "get your legs chewed off") because you want the freedom to choose your own path. Don't allow yourself to be intimidated. True friends support their friends and want the best for them. If some people in your group won't support you, you have a choice: stand firm or leave. If you choose to leave, you will make new friends who share and support your new interests.

As I write this passage, I am reminded of one of my favorite quotes written by spiritual activist Marianne Williamson:

"Our deepest fear is not that we are inadequate. Our deepest
fear is that we are powerful beyond measure. It is our light,
not our darkness that most frightens us. We ask ourselves,
'Who am I to be brilliant, gorgeous, talented, fabulous and
strong?' Actually, who are you not to be? You are a child of God.
Your playing small does not serve the world. There is nothing
enlightened about shrinking so that other people won't feel
insecure around you. We are all meant to shine, as children do.
We are born to make manifest the glory of God that is within
us. It's not just in some of us, it's in everyone. And as we let our

own light shine, we unconsciously give other people permission to do the same. And as we are liberated from our own fear, our presence automatically liberates others."

Women who shrink from the power they might gain by lifting weights can be seen in gyms everywhere. Notice the number of women doing aerobics, yoga, spinning or Pilates—everything but lifting weights. This is in spite of the fact that it's common knowledge that the shortest route to firming, toning, losing weight and preserving bone mass is through a main course of weight training with a side order of aerobics. Not that those other forms of exercise are not valuable, they're just not enough. To tone and strengthen the muscles in your body, you need to apply resistance by using a weight. As you get stronger, you must continue to incrementally increase the force applied against the muscle.

AFFIRM YOURSELF

If you have identified with any of the above beliefs about exercise, your programming may have limited your options. But you can reprogram your beliefs. You can erase the old, negative, counter-productive programming and replace it with a new positive set of messages that will help you change your attitude *and* your behavior.

To some of you this may sound too simplistic. I felt the same way, at first. Then, one morning I woke up, and instead of dragging myself out of bed wondering how I was going to make it through the day, I looked out the window and said to myself: "This is going to be a great day. I am successful, happy and healthy." And the most amazing thing happened; I did have a great day.

Without realizing it at the time, but just expecting that I

would have a great day changed the dynamic of my encounters. Feeling successful, happy and healthy made me smile and changed the response I elicited from others. My mood matched the mood of those around me.

So the next day I repeated my affirmations. And again, my day turned out even better than the last: I was offered the job I had just recently interviewed for and within a couple of weeks I could expect my first paycheck since my divorce. I was elated! Doubts that I could actually earn my own living dissolved.

Eventually affirmations became my new language. I repeated affirmations to myself throughout the day, wherever I happened to be. I stopped listening to the radio and instead repeated affirmations. I began using words like lean, fit, optimistic efficient, successful, happy, energetic, strong, vigorous, alert, powerful, certain and wise instead of sad, tired, confused, frustrated, hurried, tardy, forgetful, achy, worried and anxious. Little by little, positive, productive and encouraging beliefs replaced negative, self-defeating and demeaning beliefs.

My affirmations changed my programming; changed my body and changed my life. My wish is that affirmations will do the same for you. In the spirit of sharing, I offer you some of my favorite affirmations in the next chapter.

۲۵

CHAPTER THREE
The Power of Affirmations

"If you express your intentions, the realization of those intentions will follow." [1]

—Dr. Masaru Emoto

(Dr. Masaru Emoto is the internationally renowned Japanese scientist who has discovered that molecules of water are affected by our thoughts, words and feelings. Dr. Emoto is a graduate of the Yokohama Municipal University and the Open International University as a Doctor of Alternative Medicine.)

An affirmation is a positive statement about your self, stated in present time as though the desired change has already taken place. Affirmations can open doors and help you discover your latent qualities that you may not have otherwise recognized. When you couple an affirmation with visualization, it becomes a powerful tool for manifestation. You give your subconscious mind a command to realize a dream.

✓ I am healthy, strong and powerful.

✓ I love to work my muscles.

✓ I am learning to love what's good for me.

---

[1] Emoto, Masaru, Doctor of Alternative Medicine, *The Hidden Messages in Water* (Hillsboro, OR: Beyond Words Publishing, Inc., 2004) p.142

✓ I can do anything I set my mind to.

✓ I love to prepare nutritious food for my healthy body.

✓ When I take a deep breath I feel relaxed.

✓ I stretch to relax my muscles and release tension.

✓ I am determined to cut fat and sugar from my meals.

✓ I am beautiful, loving and kind. I love myself.

✓ I stand up for myself, even though sometimes it's difficult.

✓ Exercise is now my priority.

✓ When I'm healthy, I'm happy and I can spread happiness.

✓ I know my future health is up to me.

These are just a few of the affirmations that are most powerful for me. I usually say an affirmation while I visualize the outcome I desire. This way I envision the outcome I want and draw it towards me. For example, when I sit down to write, as I am doing now, I ask my intuition to help me find the right words to express what I'm thinking, so I can inspire others to help themselves. And the right words always come. My affirmation is: My mind is open to divine guidance. Inspiration floods my senses and I am grateful.

Nearly 25 years ago, when I first started improving my health and fitness, I thought affirmations were silly and simplistic, that I was fooling myself. But as I shared earlier, Dr. Shad Helmstetter's *What To Say When You Talk To Yourself* taught me that every thought we think, whether consciously or unconsciously, directs every feeling and action we take. His theory basically asserts: "What is out there is a reflection of what is in here."

In 1927 the brilliant scientist, Werner Karl Heisenberg, demonstrated this theory scientifically. Known as the Heisenberg Principle, one of the principles of modern physics, Heisenberg determined that, on a subatomic level, the observer's decisions affect the outcome of a physics experiment.

More recently, internationally renowned Japanese scientist Masaru Emoto has demonstrated the power of thoughts and emotions. He discovered that our thoughts, words and feelings affect molecules of water. His experiments reveal that crystals formed in frozen water show change when they receive specific thoughts or feelings. Water exposed to loving thoughts from clear springs showed brilliant and colorful snowflake patterns. By contrast, water exposed to negative thoughts formed incomplete, discolored and distorted patterns.

Dr. Emoto's book, *The Hidden Messages in Water* [2], displays many photographs of ice crystals taken via high-speed photography with both fascinating and disturbing pictures of crystals, some distorted by the negativity directed towards them, and some exposed to positive energy. For me, the most amazing picture is of the ice crystal that had been exposed to the Elvis song "Heartbreak Hotel." The crystal is split in half. Conversely, water crystals exposed to the words "love" and "gratitude" appear perfectly and brilliantly shaped.

Considering that we humans are 75 percent water, imagine what we do to our molecules when we use words like "stupid," "klutz" and "lazy." On the other hand, imagine what happens within us when we shower ourselves with words like "energetic," "smart," "healthy" and "loving."

You are everything you think you're not. All the qualities that you believe you lack to go forward, such as determination, motivation and discipline, already exist within you, waiting to be called upon, nurtured and developed. You can begin with a

---

[2] Ibid.

simple affirmation, as I once did.

I used to think that my shyness was just part of who I was, that I could never speak in public—this ability belonged only to special people. Having become a personal trainer and considering my future, I soon realized that I could not escape public speaking if I wanted to go forward in my career and increase my income.

One day I made the decision to become a fitness speaker. I began by studying successful speakers to learn what qualities they had that I lacked. To my surprise I found that the only difference between us was their speaking experience. They had gained their public speaking confidence over time by taking the risk to express themselves before audiences.

Well, I thought, I can do that too. To prepare, I began telling myself: *I am a great speaker*. I let the idea sink in for a while, and then I began to practice. I delivered mock speeches in front of mirrors and for friends. Before bedtime I visualized the exact scene, in vivid detail, of how I wanted my experience to turnout.

To make the visualization more powerful, I engaged all of my senses, so it would have a greater impact on my physiology. I stood before the microphone speaking and smiling comfortably. I heard the audience applauding with gusto and felt truly appreciated for all of my efforts. I knew they were there because they thought I had something important to say. After my speech, audience members lined up to ask questions and many thanked me for my well-delivered information.

Then I took the plunge and offered my services as a fitness speaker. Lo and behold, a community weight loss organization hired me. Even though I had months of practice under my belt, I was still terrified. But I knew I could go through it, if I could just stop shaking. So for the first three minutes I shook, while I told myself over and over, "I can do this," "I can do this." Then I settled down and finally enjoyed myself. Just as I had visualized many times, the audience loved my speech and asked lots of questions. All the hard work had paid off.

With the help of affirmations and visualizations I discovered a talent I never knew I had. What talent can you discover within yourself with the help of affirmations and visualizations? Perhaps you would like to tap into your inner athlete and uncover a yearning to become fit. If so, I invite you to join me on a walking affirmation and visualization exercise you can practice every day. Here we go.

Sit with your back supported by a pillow or wall, with hands on your lap. Close your eyes and inhale deeply through your nose. Exhale slowly through your mouth. Feel your abdomen expanding on the inhale and contracting on the exhale. Imagine yourself as you go for a walk, describing what you see, hear and feel.

Walking every day in nature is my new goal. But, if I'm unable to go outside, I will find an alternative. I can climb the stairs in my house or simply walk from my front door to the back porch and back. I am on a mission to improve my health and feel better about myself. I deserve 30 minutes just for me. I am worth it. So here I go, out the door. It's really lovely out here. The sun is shining; a soft breeze caresses my skin. Birds are singing and oh, look, a tiny squirrel there in front of me. I take a deep breath and pick up the pace a bit. I feel my heart pumping a little faster. I keep my faster pace for a little while and then slow it down again. I read once that you can burn more calories when you alternate between fast and slow, rather than keeping a steady rhythm throughout. I'm really enjoying being out here, feeling my body move, using my muscles, perspiring a bit, taking in fresh air. I didn't think I could go this far, but here I am, going further than ever before. I can tell my body likes this walk; it's moving a lot smoother now than when I started. I'm going to do this every day. I can't wait to come back here tomorrow.

Practice this walking meditation every day for a week. Your subconscious will register your desire to be healthy and one day without even thinking about it, you will surprise yourself. You will just get up and take off for a walk.

CREATING YOUR OWN AFFIRMATIONS

For the first few days after you begin your own process, pay careful attention to your thoughts and words. Don't judge, simply listen to both your negative and positive self-talk. At the end of the day, make a list of your negative statements. These might include statements like: "I can't do that," "I hate that," "That's impossible for me," "Never in a million years will I be able to do that" and so on. Once you have a list of your negative self-talk, change each statement to a positive one. Keep making your list on a daily basis, transforming each negative statement to a positive one. Soon, you'll begin to catch yourself as the negative words leave your mouth. When this happens you will soon be able to make the "negative-to-positive" connection instantly.

I would like to share with you some of my past negative self-talk and the changes I made. Following my list, I will provide you with a blank page where you can write your own negative messages and make necessary changes.

My former negative self-talk	My new positive self-talk
I never look as good as she does.	I'm happy with the way I look.
If I say what I think, they won't like me.	I feel good when I express what I really think and feel.
I could never do that. I just don't have that in me.	I am learning to challenge myself in every way.
I hate how I look.	I'm looking better every day.
I hate myself for not speaking up.	It's difficult to speak up, but I'm doing it.
It's no use; this is how I was born.	I can change anything about myself one step at a time.
I'm always late, but it's not my fault.	I'm getting ready earlier so I can be on time.
I'm used to eating this way.	I'm willing to try new foods for my health's sake.
I hate my nose.	I love my nose.
Why is my skin breaking out at my age?	I'm grateful for my clear skin.
I love to have desserts after every meal.	I'm learning to like fruit instead of sugary sweets.

Now I invite you to make a list of your own negative self-talk. Think back to yesterday. Did you make any statements like "I'm stupid," "I'm forgetful," "I can't do anything right," "I'm getting sloppier by the minute," "he hates me," "I'm always late," "I hate myself for doing that" and so on?

If so, list those statements below. Be honest with yourself. We can't change what we refuse to acknowledge. When finished, make the corresponding changes in the positive self-talk column.

Invest a few minutes each day on this exercise. Once you begin to acknowledge and take responsibility for what you say when you talk to yourself, you'll begin to see how negativity diminishes your value. Armed with this new awareness, you can now choose to address yourself with the respect and honor that you deserve.

Your negative self-talk	Your new positive self-talk

You can also make affirmation cards to put in places where you spend a lot of time, like your bathroom, bedside table, kitchen counter, dashboard or on your computer's desktop. One of the best times for affirmations is just before bedtime. By giving your subconscious mind clear and direct instructions, you create your future.

For me, affirmations have become mantras that I repeat to myself in moments of silence. I don't want my mind to be idle, to allow negative thoughts to intrude and take root.

Once you focus on yourself, begin to focus on the self-talk of those around you. Again, don't judge, simply pay attention. You will become more aware of the kinds of thoughts you allow to take up space in your consciousness. You will no longer mindlessly absorb negative messages that can influence your life decisions.

If you don't see changes right away, remember that it takes time to change thought patterns that have existed for many years—perhaps for most of your life. As much as 78 percent of our thoughts are negative, counter-productive and self-defeating—all the more important to daily reinforce positive messages by repeating affirmations. The more often you tell yourself you're committed and disciplined, the sooner you will believe it. Once the belief is in place, you have already become the person you want to be. After that, anything is possible.

I owe Louise L. Hay, author of *You Can Heal Your Life* [3], a debt of gratitude for having introduced me to the practice of affirmations. When I was going through a difficult time with my eyes. I had been told by my ophthalmologist that I needed a corneal transplant. But I believed that the natural healing techniques I had just discovered could restore my sight. I didn't want surgery.

[3] Hay, Louise L., *You Can Heal Your Life* (Carlsbad, CA: Hay House, Inc., 2005)

I practiced eye regenerating exercises and affirmations every day for years, and eventually my sight improved. I never had the surgery. Twenty years later, I still say my eye affirmations: my eyes are perfectly clear, focused and sharp.

ℰℐᴐ

CHAPTER FOUR
Emotional Cleansing & Self-Esteem

"I see the process of communication we have demonstrated, the flow of information through the whole organism, as evidence that the body is the actual outward manifestation, in physical space, of the mind." [1]

—Candace B. Pert, Ph. D.

(When she wrote her book, , Candace Pert was research professor in the Department of Physiology and Biophysics, Georgetown University Medical Center, Washington D. C.)

W e all share a human instinct to seek pleasure and avoid pain, including painful recollections. Freud called it the "pleasure principle." To distance ourselves from our painful realities we repress our emotions, rationalize our behavior and distort past events. Denial, the most common defense mechanism of choice, causes us to unconsciously ignore painful and distressing facts about ourselves and others. We look away from the pain for fear of *feeling* the pain.

But pain that we do not explore, express or resolve cannot be

---

[1] Pert, Candace B., Ph.D., *Molecules of Emotion: The Science Behind Mind-Body Medicine* (New York: Simon & Schuster, 1999) p. 187.

repressed forever. Instead it leaks out in destructive behaviors, physical illnesses and interpersonal conflict. The following fictional stories illustrate how painful experiences left unexplored and unresolved prevent people from realizing their dreams. We all have a story to tell. Most of our shame centers around problems with overeating, body image and neck and back pain. All of these themes are universal in nature. Being that we all want to be loved, when we encounter criticism, it damages our sense of self.

(From Marcia, a 55 year-old housewife) (I am EE.)

EE: "You told me on the phone that you need to exercise because you want to lose weight, so let's talk about your eating habits first. Do you cook at home or eat out?"

Marcia: "I eat out a lot. But when I eat out I just play with my food, I never eat it. Later when I get home, I go straight to the refrigerator and eat everything in sight. I stuff myself and then I feel sick. I don't like myself when I do that."

This 55 year-old woman had a serious eating condition she would need to explore. Her repressed guilt and shame triggered her overeating. To be free of their control, she had to explore the sources of these emotions. When did these shameful feelings first manifest themselves? How old was she? What were the circumstances? Who was present at the time?

(From Jen, a 25-year-old young woman living at home)

EE: "Why do you want to start lifting weights?"

Jen: "I want to change everything about myself. I hate the way I look."

EE: "I can understand that you want to be fit, but you are beautiful as you are. Do you know how many people would love to look the way you do? You could be a model. Why do you think you hate the way you look?"

Jen: "I don't know. Maybe it's because I heard a lot of criticisms when I was little, and that made me feel bad about myself. "

This truly beautiful young woman hated herself and thought she was ugly. From a very young age she had been exposed to negative messages about her appearance that she had internalized and come to believe about herself.

(From Jane, a 35 year-old high-school teacher)

EE: "I don't know for sure that there's anything I can do to help you heal your back pain, but let's see what we can do. We'll start with some stretches, deep breathing and light weights. Every night before you go to bed, I want you to read over this list of affirmations. Then close your eyes and imagine your back pain diminishing. Believe that healing is possible. I also want you to read this little book on the mind-body connection, the link between stress and back pain."

Jane: "Okay, I've got to get rid of this pain."

When I asked Jane if she could pinpoint the source of her stress, she mentioned being unhappy with her job and sitting for long hours at the computer and in the classroom. I gave Jane the book *Healing Back Pain*[2] by Dr. John E. Sarno, professor of Clinical Rehabilitation Medicine at the New York University School of Medicine. Dr. Sarno's book proposes that anxiety and repressed anger trigger muscle spasms, and that our lower back particularly suffers when we experience mental and emotional stress.

Jane's body manifested severe back pain from sitting for long hours, but also from her frustration and disappointment over her job situation. Dr. Candace B. Pert, a brilliant scientist,

---

[2] Sarno, John E., M.D., *Healing Back Pain: The Mind Body Connection* (New York: Warner Books, Inc., 1991)

substantiated the liberating fact that the mind impacts the body, a message that continues to evolve and enhance understanding of the direct, unified relationship between mind and body.

In her landmark book, *Molecules of Emotion,* Dr. Pert reveals through her pioneering research how our thoughts and emotions affect our health. She describes how the chemicals produced within our bodies form an interconnecting network of information that links mind and body. The mind creates the flow of information, as it moves among the cells, organs and systems of the body. Mind doesn't dominate body, it *becomes* body—body and mind are one.

Troubles in the mind carried over time can impact our lives and stunt our evolution. In his book entitled *Living the Truth: Transform Your Life Through the Power of Insight and Honesty,* psychiatrist Keith Ablow states that the pain of suffering through abuse, neglect, loss of a loved one or growing up with an alcoholic, must be resolved if we are to heal from such wounding. As long as we avoid coming to terms with the truth rooted in our past, we cannot live authentic lives and become who we were meant to be.

The psychological conflict created by unresolved issues from our past drives our destructive behaviors. We overeat, we abuse drugs or alcohol and we punish ourselves through neglect. To find our inner power, Dr. Ablow suggests, "we must come to terms with the truth rooted in our past—our greatest source of power."[3]

SURRENDER

I am a perfect example of someone who could not get past

---

[3] Ablow, Keith, *Living the Truth: Transform Your Life Through the Power of Insight and Honesty* (New York: Little, Brown and Company, 2007)

failure and pain until I'd resolved my psychological distress. As I mentioned earlier, my old life was riddled with chaos and illnesses, including two divorces, cancer, near-blindness and, finally, near-bankruptcy. I had never made the connection between my calamities and my painful past. Instead, I blamed everything on bad luck.

One day, after my last divorce, when I was feeling desolate and rejected by life, I sat and truly thought about my life for the very first time. Until then, reflection had been a menacing stranger. Now, questions flooded my thinking. Why had my life taken the course it had? Why hadn't I been able to cultivate a normal life like other people I knew?

Overwhelmed with so many questions, I addressed whoever could hear me: *I need help. Please tell me what I need to do and I'll do it. I haven't done well on my own. I need guidance.*

With those words, I surrendered my old ways to God—my anger, my guilt, my shame and fears. As if in answer, a strong urge to be healthy rushed through my body. I knew then that if I was going to go forward as a new person and create a new life, I needed to be healthy and strong. The next day I joined a gym and started lifting weights.

Proper lifting requires proper breathing, and through the breath I discovered the connection between my mind and my body. I remember clearly the moment I first became aware of my negative self-talk. As I exhaled on the exertion of a particular shoulder move, I "heard" the thought *you can't do it,* pop into my head. Surprised that I actually was able to differentiate positive from negative, I immediately changed "can't" to "I can". Before that moment, I had never given the commands coming from my mind any attention and yet they were directing my every move while also creating my reality.

My life changed that moment in the gym when I transformed my negative inner statement into a positive one. From that day forward, my affirmations continuously voice and deliver positive and encouraging commands that guide my feelings and actions toward the health, happiness and success that I deserve and desire.

KNOW THYSELF

While I continued training, I kept searching for answers to my many questions. I read countless self-help books and wrote about my childhood experiences growing up in an alcoholic home. Through this process I released the withheld emotions I had carried for so long that had kept me chained to the past. I now felt free, and healed. Writing also brought the child I had been close to my heart. I now cherish and love her, instead of rejecting and despising her. I now feel deep and abiding compassion for the little girl I was and who will always be with me.

We all carry our inner child within us.

In time, I brought the pieces of my life together. Life now makes sense. I realize that when I hide my feelings to protect myself from painful and frightening experiences, I also shut out other parts of myself: my creativity, my spontaneity, my joy and my daring nature.

In unearthing and shedding light on these neglected parts of myself I have become whole. I am now complete—compassionate and confident that I can choose what is best for me. I can now parent myself, giving myself the love, nurture and care that I had lacked as a child. My journey towards wholeness has allowed me to nourish and strengthen my self-esteem.

Once I accepted the truth of my past, sharing that truth became one of my greatest sources of power. It awakened intimacy in my life not only with my sons, but also everyone else. I can now tell my story without fear or shame, knowing it is simply another story of the human being's universal search for the true self.

DEPRESSION AND ALIENATION

During my senior year of high school I gained 25 pounds.

I weighed 115 pounds when I arrived at boarding school and 140 when I left. I ate constantly to soothe my sadness, fears and insecurities. Only food held my interest. Every afternoon after classes I sat in the schoolyard with half a dozen chocolate candy bars and ate every single one of them.

Carrying 25 pounds more than my normal weight increased my feelings of unworthiness and gave me another reason to hate myself. I dressed with the specific purpose of hiding my despised body parts: long sleeves to hide my fat arms and pleats to hide my big stomach.

My negative self-talk and worldview fueled my depression. I focused on the negative side of life and expected failure to befall me at every turn. I misinterpreted every comment addressed to or about me, opening my wounds and proving to myself that life meant suffering.

Through my journey toward wholeness I learned that an absence of spiritual connection had been for years at the root of my depression. My depression grew out of my hunger for connection to my deepest self, my innermost thoughts, feelings and emotions. Only through surrender to God could I dissolve my depression and find my true self.

Many of us lose this connection to our deepest self as a response to trauma experienced in childhood. The link between depression and childhood trauma has been well documented in family dynamics and many of us have experienced firsthand some form of trauma arising out of emotional, physical or sexual abuse in addition to divorce, poverty and addiction.

In response to the pains and stresses of growing up in difficult environments where we may have felt rejected, humiliated or neglected, we learned to repress our thoughts, feelings and emotions for fear of being ostracized.

"What's wrong with you, why are you sad?" "You have no reason to be unhappy." "Don't get angry at me, or else." Sound familiar? These messages confused us and sent a clear message that our true feelings and emotions were unacceptable. To keep our place within the family, we shut down our true feelings and replaced them with pleasing ones. As children we could not risk defiance, as our very livelihood depended on compliance.

I responded with sadness, fear and anger to growing up in the midst of the abuse and chaos typically associated with an alcoholic home. Later these feelings developed into my depression.

For many years I experienced symptoms of clinical depression: feelings of alienation (I was a stranger to myself and others), helplessness (I was overwhelmed by deep sadness), and hopelessness (things could be worse, so accept what you've got), indecisiveness (without a sense of self, I had no concrete knowledge of what I liked, stood for or believed in).

Sad, angry and anxious, but unable to fully experience and express what I was feeling, I tortured myself by ruminating for hours, sometimes days, for not saying what I should have said, or doing what I should have done. I hated myself for being such a coward. Waves of sadness followed episodes of defeat. Eventually I ended where I started, convinced that I deserved my miserable situation. Nothing ever changed, and the next day the cycle would repeat itself all over again.

The tragedy of depression is that while we're in the midst of it, it's almost impossible to recognize that we're suffering an illness, a mental disorder that's not normal, and that we need help.

When left untreated, depression can lead to chronic diseases, like cancer.

In her book entitled, *The Type C Connection, The Behavioral Links to Cancer and Your Health*,[4] Dr. Lydia Temoshok, writes that Type C Behavior, a particular coping mechanism found common in many of her cancer patients, is linked to cancer risk.

Type C Behavior is the depressive state of mind that I described earlier as my own, the inability to express anger, even recognize that we're angry or convey any emotion at all. Passive and appeasing in personal relationships, the cancer patients in Dr. Temoshok's study self-sacrificed to the extreme, always putting others' needs before their own. She based her findings on interviews with more than 150 melanoma patients, three-fourths of whom exhibited the Type C Behavior pattern.

I read Dr. Temoshok's book because I wanted to know why I had gotten cancer. When I read her description of the Type C Behavior personality, I recognized my old self. I knew then that my cancer had not come out of nowhere nor by chance. Even though I realized that my behavior had contributed to my developing cancer, I did not, however, feel guilty, as I understood that my previous choices had been made unconsciously. To the contrary, this new information empowered me. I knew I could never get cancer again. My new assertive, nurturing, loving and emotionally expressive personality insured me against illness by perpetually boosting my immune system.

[4] Temoshok, Lydia, Ph.D., and Henry Dreher, *The Type C Connection, The Behavioral Links to Cancer and Your Health* (New York: Random House, 1992)

If you're suffering from depression, if you're unhappy with your life, feel trapped in a relationship or believe that as miserable as your situation is, it's better than nothing, seek help first and foremost. Joining a group class, lifting weights, writing about your feelings and other initiatives that may spark your interest can give you just the lift you need.

Studies have shown that especially expressing feelings and emotions through the writing process can boost immunity and enhance overall health. Divulging long-held secrets offers a tremendous sense of freedom and renewed vigor and vitality. We don't realize, while in the midst of our depression, that our bodies' suffer from the extra tension of keeping secrets. Our alienation from ourselves can only heal by opening our hearts, by acknowledging our pain to ourselves and to others.

Some of you may be cringing at the thought of facing your childhood pain for fear of being misinterpreted as intending to cast blame. I know I did, and for many years I suffered needlessly. This process is not about blame, but forgiveness. Our caretakers had limited knowledge of proper child-rearing practices. This is an intergenerational problem reaching back countless generations.

Of great importance, says Dr. Temoshok, is to realize that there are no *negative* emotions. Anger, sadness and fear are not toxic unless repression becomes a habit or we identify with the emotion and it engulfs us. Their purpose is a noble one, a positive sign from our bodies, that something must change to relieve our distress.

Expressing my full-range of emotions calls me to daily diligence and has become a necessary and worthy mission. "If the feelings cannot be experienced, discharged or properly managed," writes Dr. Temoshok, "a biological imperative is blocked. The long-term consequence is mind-body imbalance."

We all know the Type A personalities who vent their rage outwardly. They scream, hit, insult. Type C's vent their anger inwardly. We self-sacrifice, self-neglect and blame ourselves for others' mistakes, the reason depression is also known as "anger turned inward".

Dr. Temoshok explains that the person who chronically resists expressing needs and feelings will suffer a myriad of harmful consequences. "Whoever loses touch with primary emotions, also loses touch with physical sensations," she affirms, "When you can't feel anger, fear or sadness, eventually you have a hard time feeling anything." Emotional numbness also blocks sensations of physical pain and exhaustion while psychological needs remain neglected.

According to government statistics, up to 80 percent of people who go to doctors suffer from an underlying depression (National Healthcare Quality Report, 2003). Thirty percent of women are depressed, and 41 percent are too embarrassed to seek help.

Studies show a link between depression and a host of other diseases besides cancer, from osteoporosis, heart attacks, loss of vision, certain forms of cancer and diabetes.[5]

So what is the cure for depression? To date, the most common treatments, antidepressants and cognitive behavior therapy, are not long-term solutions.

Dr. Temoshok's program for transformation recommends learning to manage anger effectively, becoming assertive, expressing feelings and emotion and practicing mind-body relaxation exercises to relieve stress and anxiety. Mind, body and

---

[5] http://www.upliftprogram.com/article_together.html

emotions must be integrally addressed.

To that list I would add exercise. Exercise became my first line of defense in my quest for healing. Exercise flooded my mind with endorphins, the "feel good" chemicals that bathed my body with hope and optimism, while cognitive behavior therapy helped me to change my thinking patterns and behaviors.

Cognitive behavior therapy is based on the belief that our thoughts cause our feelings and behaviors. If we want to feel and act better, we must create thoughts that are productive and uplifting. This concept, covered in Chapter 2, Reprogramming Outdated Beliefs, empowers us to manage difficult situations, people and events.

My depression began to lift when I began to lift weights and develop my body. I felt my inner power seep into my muscles and I regained confidence in my ability to achieve whatever goal I set for myself. Today I am proud of who I am and what I've accomplished. I radiate with aliveness and love—the true meaning of success.

I have not been depressed for 25 years. Just as I believe I will never again have cancer, I believe my depressed days are over. Today I am the opposite of who I was then, down to my cellular core. My prayer for guidance and my eventual spiritual connection saved me, along with physical exercise and my own brand of cognitive behavior. Together these healed my brain, emotions and body—permanently.

Unless we know who we are and why we do the things we do, we continue to repeat self-defeating and destructive behaviors. On the path to health and longevity "to know thyself" is essential. It is the first step towards developing self-esteem. Once you value yourself, you can nurture yourself without interruption, without suffering flashes of painful experiences from the past, over and over again, demanding to be resolved.

"If you bring forth what is within you, what you bring forth will save you. If you do not bring forth what is within you, what you do not bring forth will destroy you."

—Jesus Christ, The Gospel of St. Thomas

REPARENTING OURSELVES

I believe that our unhappiness comes not from the absence of love in the past, but rather from the love we fail to give to ourselves in the present.

What are some of the blessings you wish you'd received in your childhood but did not? Was it emotional connection, a loving touch? Was it validation of your feelings, confirmation of your ideas? Or was it encouragement in the face of despair?

If you experienced a childhood in which no one pointed to the stars and told you that you could go there, the good news is that now you can—*because you can take yourself there.* And what better way to begin that journey than to start taking care of your mind, body and spirit?

Enrich your mind with inspirational affirmations, exercise your body and spend time reflecting on your behavior. This new process of self-care will help you to connect with your true self— your visions, aspirations and dreams for both your body and your life. Every step you take from now on can lead you to your true essence—your strength, your beauty and your courage.

BUILDING SELF-ESTEEM

Self-esteem simply means to esteem the self. Do you value yourself enough to do the right thing for yourself in all areas of your life? Do you take care of your needs, wants and desires? Do you follow through on your commitments to change whenever you see an area that needs correcting? Ask yourself these questions to begin to put your self first.

You are the most important person in your life. When you respect yourself, you respect others; when you love yourself, you can love others; when you take care of yourself first, you can take care of others. Your health is the most important thing in your life, because without it, what do you have?

Money, career and status won't save you when you get sick.

Self-esteem is the key to happiness and well-being. When you have self-esteem you feel deserving of happiness. You have self-respect and care for your health—body, mind and spirit.

To assess your level of self-esteem, ask yourself a few questions: Do you walk through your life projecting the pleasure and joy you take in being alive? Do you express gratitude often? Do you feel free to express what you think and feel? Do you enjoy giving and receiving compliments? Are you receptive to new ideas and concepts? Are you comfortable being assertive?

If so, self-esteem manifests itself in your life. When you exhibit these qualities, you are comfortable within your own skin. You feel relaxed about who you are, rather than being at war with yourself.

When you struggle with self-esteem, you may notice a "mismatch" between your beliefs and your actions. If you hear yourself say: "Oh, I know I should exercise, but I just can't get myself to do it" or "I don't know why I can't follow through on my plan to eat healthy," stop for a moment. Breathe. Reflect. Recommit.

In my experience, when we say, "I don't know why I do this or don't do that," what we're really saying is, "I'm not ready to take responsibility for myself." I heard author and spiritual lecturer Marianne Williamson, whose poem I quoted in Chapter 3, respond to an audience member who had answered her question with "I don't know why," by saying, "You are not allowed to say 'I don't know'. So let me ask the question again." When she did, the woman answered with the truth.

A commitment to awareness is one of the first steps toward self-esteem. Become aware of your thoughts and words. Remember, they have tremendous creative power. When you tune into the messages you give yourself, commit to your healthy lifestyle and align your thoughts and behavior, self-acceptance will follow. You will look in the mirror and be satisfied. Your new sense of responsibility will foster further positive change.

Become an independent thinker, practice awareness, sit in reflection, clarify your values and assert your convictions. And, if you feel the need, write the story of your life. Now, you can develop a clearer understanding of your outdated beliefs, learn how to reprogram your thinking through the use of affirmations and reflect on the possible sources of unhealthy behaviors.

It's time to get to work on building your new body. Building strength, in itself, will help to boost your self-esteem.

છ૭

CHAPTER FIVE
The Vibrant Health Workout

"Create a healthy, strong body early, and then simply maintain it. It is much easier to maintain than to build when you are in your later years." [1]

—Dr. Walter M. Bortz, II

(Former co-chairman of the American Medical Association's Task Force on Aging, and former president of the American Geriatric Society.)

THOUGHTS ON GETTING STARTED

Begin with the basics. The following workout schedule is for beginners. However, by increasing both the number of repetitions and sets, and also the weight incrementally, as you get stronger, the workout can serve any level of fitness.

After training for more than two decades, I continue to perform these exercises on a regular basis. Of course, I lift much more weight today than I did when I began my fitness program 25 years ago.

My Vibrant Health Workout addresses major muscle groups with simple exercises that can be performed with a minimum of

[1] Bortz II, Walter M., M.D. and Stickrod, Randall, *The Roadmap to 100* (New York: Palgrave MacMillan, 2010) p.115.

equipment: incline bench, barbell, dumbbells and ankle weights.

If you don't have a bench, you can use pillows to elevate your chest, shoulders and head (see page 70). Doing chest exercises on an inclined surface will strengthen and tone the muscles that support the breast above the nipple area.

You can do this workout either at home or at the gym, so there are no excuses!

My Vibrant Health Workout has benefited 20 year olds to 80 year olds, but check with your doctor before starting this or any other exercise program.

Consider hiring a personal trainer to get you started. Weight training can be overwhelming for someone who has never lifted a weight before. A trainer can facilitate your learning process and speed progress. Look for a trainer who teaches from experience not only book knowledge. Make sure they look fit!

A qualified and experienced trainer can teach you proper form and breathing patterns, help modify exercises to meet your personal needs and encourage you through the initial hurdles. Hire a confident, straightforward trainer who will tell you the truth. You don't need a chatty, social partner. You need a trainer who will say what needs saying, for example: negative thoughts and self-criticism can seriously derail your progress toward fitness.

You can also train yourself. If you are well motivated, you can teach yourself the principles of weight training. You can start with this book and then expand your knowledge. Read all you can on the subject from different sources.

I started with Rachel McLish's book, *Flex Appeal.* I admired her toned, not overly muscular body. Once I learned everything I could from Rachel's book, I continued reading. I subscribed to fitness magazines and read them thoroughly not only about lifting weights, but also about nutrition, motivation, meditation and how to change negative patterns.

You can do the same and become your own coach.

Pace yourself. If you have been inactive for years, you may suffer from a decreased range of motion, joint problems and/or cardiovascular deficiencies. If any one or all of these is true, you'll need to be very patient with yourself.

I have seen many people give up because they couldn't get their bodies into the right position on their first try, or because they became exhausted within five minutes of working out.

I once trained Margie, a 65-year-old woman who had never exercised before. Fifteen minutes into her workout, she wanted to quit. I coached her to deep breathe and relax. I then divided her routine into manageable, five-minute sections following each with a few minutes of deep breathing and stretching. Eventually, Margie could tolerate a whole hour of exercise without becoming panicked or discouraged. Fifteen years later, she's still working out. She looks great and, more important, she feels wonderful!

Panic can also set in when a woman has never played sports and experienced the "flushed face" of exertion. Instead of interpreting as natural the rush of blood that creates a desirable, rosy facial glow, some women see this as a negative experience.

Joan, a client who was just learning to squat, became flushed. Her face had turned red with the rush of blood to her head. When she saw herself in the mirror, she panicked. "I have to stop, I have to stop, I need to sit!" she cried. I told her to sit and breathe. I then explained to her that what she felt was perfectly normal. Unfortunately, Joan had been taught early on, that flushing was dangerous. Her mother's admonitions to "sit" when she ran into the house from the yard with a red face still had power over her, even though long an adult. When she learned that her flushing was nothing more than blood rushing to her skin's surface, a natural consequence of exertion, she could resume her workout.

These two situations of the many I have encountered illustrate how facts and encouragement have helped my clients continue their exercise programs. In such situations, having a knowledgeable, supportive personal trainer can be invaluable.

Using free weights vs. machines. All of my training, both personal and professional, is done with free weights with the exception of the leg extension machine that strengthens the quadriceps and hamstring muscles. Free weights are inexpensive, versatile and easily stored. But training with barbells and dumbbells yields superior overall strength. Free weights are simply more effective than machines for developing smaller synergistic (helping) muscles and stabilizer muscles. Also, when using free weights, limbs work independently of each other, instead of the strong limb doing all of the work.

I tested machines early in my training career, but soon realized I could not develop the desired muscle, unless I switched to free weights. Machines, designed to fit *average* size bodies, did not fit my 5'2" frame and cut down on my range of motion. Knowing the essential importance of range of motion, I switched to free weights and never looked back.

WEIGHT TRAINING GUIDELINES

Let's start with a few definitions:

Reps: One complete round of lifting and lowering of weight.

Sets: A number of reps performed in a single exercise.

Frequency: How often you work out per week. (I recommend two to three times per week, with one day of rest in between.)

Duration: How long you work out during one session. (I recommend 20 to 40 to 60 minutes, depending on your fitness level.)

Range of Motion: The distance and direction a joint can move to its full potential.

Warm-up. Readies your body for action. You can either breathe consciously while walking in place or bicycling for four to five minutes to send oxygen to your heart, your working muscles and your brain.

Focus on form. In the beginning stages of weight training, intensity should take a backseat to proper form and technique. As a beginner, you need to concentrate on the proper execution of each exercise—the coordination of lifting and lowering of weight with the breathing pattern. I recommend starting with 20 repetitions of each exercise with two- or three-pound weights. (The "rule of ten" refers to using a weight with which you can do no more than ten repetitions, but this is applicable to intermediate and advanced trainees, not beginners.) First, master technique. Then, increase the weight load incrementally to maintain new peak strength. If you begin with a weight that is too heavy, you will struggle to lift the weight and more likely forget about form, perhaps even suffering an injury.

Lift for one, lower for two. Lift for a count of one, lower for a count of two. Resist as you lower the weight. Do not suddenly drop the weight, or swing it. Handle the weight in a smooth, controlled manner. Do not lock your joints (elbows, knees and shoulders). Such constant pressure can eventually cause injury.

Time between sets. The amount of time you spend between sets depends on level of experience. From one to three minutes, or as long as it takes for a slow, deep breath is long enough.

Take care of your joints. It takes longer for joints to

strengthen, compared to muscles. For the first few months, do higher repetitions with lighter weights (20 repetitions of each exercise with three-to-five pound weights). This method will give your joints time to strengthen and to catch up to your muscles. Due to disuse, your joints may suffer from a short supply of the synovial fluid that lubricates the joints, acts as a shock absorber and nourishes the surrounding cartilage. Take it easy!

Pay attention to breathing: Inhale on the extension, the lowering phase of the movement. Exhale on the contraction, the lifting phase of the movement. Be mindful not to hold your breath (for even as long as eight seconds). This could cause fainting. Holding your breath increases internal pressure in the chest and abdomen. Always exhale as fully as you inhale.

Drink lots of water: Drink water before, during and after exercise. Proper hydration helps your body stay cool, lubricates your joints and helps rebound from your workouts. Dehydration can cause cramping, dizziness and nausea.

Easy does it. If any exercise in My Vibrant Health Workout feels uncomfortable, skip it and go to the next exercise. Concentrate first on the ones that are easy, and then later go back to the ones you found harder. Try each of them, one by one. No one exercise fits all.

Stretch between sets. Stretching increases your range of motion and allows your muscles to generate more force throughout all movements.

Try a squat substitute. If you suffer from knee, ankle, lower-back or hip problems, substitute the Glute Press or Donkey Kick (see page 85) for the squat.

Concentrate and focus: When you work out, you get to know your body. When you begin to connect mind to muscle, you *read* your body and respond to its signals when stress or injury has caused it to lose its balance. Paying attention to the signal prevents or reduces damage and soon you will respond at the very first sign of discomfort. People disconnected from their bodies tend to ignore blaring signs of distress and react only after it's too late.

Engage power of your mind. Mind and muscle are one. To help you speed this mind-to-muscle process, I recommend that you invest in an anatomy book, such as the classic *Gray's Anatomy*. As you train, this will give you a visual reference for tuning in to the muscle you're working. When you prepare to perform a particular exercise, turn to the drawing for the particular muscle you plan to work. Keep that picture in your mind as you perform the set number of repetitions. *Feel* the stretching and contracting of the muscle as you move it through its full range of motion and breathe simultaneously. Using visual imagery will support training with more precision, inviting you to become intimate with your body while preventing injury and speeding muscle growth.

Walk for cardiovascular endurance. Aerobic fitness enhances the efficiency of both the respiratory and circulatory system. It also increases your muscles' ability to utilize fat as a source of energy. If you are a beginner, walk as far as you can, as fast as you can and as often as you can. Breathe and drink water. It's important to sustain sufficient hydration. Gradually, increase both intensity and duration of your working regimen. For a basic, minimum level aerobic benefit, walk for 30 minutes three to four times a week. Depending on the state of your health, walk at a low to moderate level of intensity.

Low intensity would be how you feel when walking from your car to the grocery store. You're purposely attentive, concentrating on getting to your destination. You can speak comfortably. Your heartbeat is slightly elevated. Moderate intensity is how you feel when walking in the park for exercise. You exert yourself more and breathe a little harder. You may feel the need to inhale more deeply.

Cool down. Cool down for five to ten minutes at the end of each of your exercise sessions. After a resistance training session, lactic acid accumulates in the muscles, causes discomfort and reduces performance. Light stretching or gentle aerobics after a workout can help your body eliminate the lactic acid and reduce muscles soreness.

Recovery. Pay attention to your body. If something hurts, back off from your workout. Muscle soreness after a workout is normal; pain is not. Sometimes ice, heat and stretching can take care of minor discomforts, but if what you feel is real pain, see a doctor.

Refuel. Refueling your body with protein and carbohydrates within one hour after your workout restores and rebuilds your muscles. A rule of thumb is the 1:4 ratio—one part protein, four parts complex carbohydrates. I enjoy a recovery drink that contains 10 grams of protein and 40 grams of carbohydrates, along with Vitamins C and E to help reduce muscle soreness and promote muscle repair and growth. Within two hours after a workout, it's best to have a small, healthy meal. I have a small piece of fish with rice or a spinach taco.

Rest. Muscles need rest to recover and rebuild. Since our muscles actually grow on their day of rest, we don't want to work the same muscle two days in a row.

Massage between workouts. I believe that massage is a necessary complement to a workout regimen. Massage can help reduce injury, improve range of motion and eliminate toxins. It's especially important for those of us over 50 who may be taking up exercise for the first time. Massage can help heal the wear and tear that naturally accompanies strenuous exercise. Though I only began treating myself to massage after I suffered an injury, since then I have one regularly and consider it a necessity. After a massage my body always feels more flexible and fluid.

Your workout schedule: The following workout schedule is very simple. It consists of 16 exercises that will work all of your major muscle groups. My best advice is to get very comfortable with these particular exercises. You want *to know* and to *feel* the muscles as you work them, and then to incrementally *increase* the weight. *You must tax the muscle with enough weight to force the muscle to grow and strengthen.* If you do this consistently, you can build a body that will take you into your 90s and beyond with resiliency and stamina.

If you stay truly committed to your Vibrant Health Workout schedule, my experience tells me that in only a short time, you will begin to feel stronger, more energetic and generally more confident. Being fit will open a whole new world of possibility for you. I never could have imagined that 25 years later I would still enjoy working out as much as I did when I started. But here I am, still amazed at what exercise does for me. My peace of mind, happiness and success in all that I do depends on my daily exercise. My wish is that you too will discover the same pleasures and benefits.

WEIGHT TRAINING WORKOUT SCHEDULE

Warm-up: 10 minute treadmill walk or march in place

Flexibility: 5 minutes of light stretching

CHEST	Reps	Sets	Weight
Chest Press	15-20	1	
Chest Flyes	15-20	1	
SHOULDERS			
Press	15-20	1	
Front Lift	15-20	1	
Lateral Lift	15-20	1	
Rear Deltoid	15-20	1	
ARMS & BACK			
Back Rows	15-20	1	
Biceps Curl	15-20	1	
Triceps Extension	15-20	1	
Lying Triceps	15-20	1	
ABDOMINALS			
Crunch	20-25	1	
GLUTES & LEGS			
Squat / Donkey Kick	15-20	1	
Dead Lift (Power Lift)	15-20	1	
Quad Extension (seated)	20-25	1	
Hamstring Curl	20-25	1	
Calf Raise	20-25	1	
Inner Thigh	20-25	1	
Outer Thigh	20-25	1	
Alternate legs	20-25	1	
Cool Down: 5 minutes of light/moderate stretching.			

I have provided you with a blank workout schedule so you can fill it in with your own information. You can record the number of repetitions, sets and the amount of weight you use. Keeping a schedule will strengthen your commitment.

YOUR PERSONAL WORKOUT SCHEDULE

CHEST	Reps	Sets	Weight
Chest Press			
Chest Flyes			
SHOULDERS			
Press			
Front Lift			
Lateral Lift			
Rear Deltoid			
ARMS & BACK			
Back Rows			
Biceps Curl			
Triceps Extension			
Lying Triceps			
ABDOMINALS			
Crunch			
GLUTES & LEGS			
Squat / Donkey Kick			
Dead Lift (Power Lift)			
Quad Extension (seated)			
Hamstring Curl			
Calf Raise			
Inner Thigh			
Outer Thigh			
Alternate legs			
Cool Down: 5 minutes of light/moderate stretching.			

VIBRANT HEALTH WORKOUT

The Vibrant Health Workout includes focused exercises for the chest, shoulders, arms and back, abdominals, glutes and legs, alternate legs and stretching.

CHEST EXERCISES

(pectoralis major)

The *pectoralis* major muscle is responsible for keeping the arm attached to the body and is essential for proper posture. Beginner women should do a good portion of all chest exercises on an incline surface to tone the *upper* pecs. This is the part of the chest muscle that supports the breast. It is also the part of the chest more readily seen.

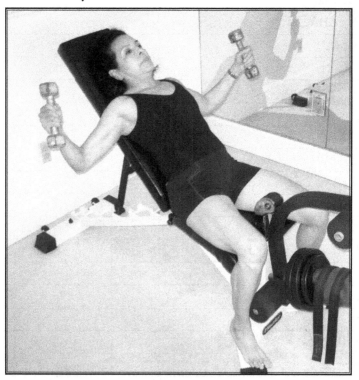

Figure 1 - Chest Flye

Figure 1 - Chest Flyes. (This exercise works the major muscles of the chest with emphasis on the outer portion.) Hold the dumbbells directly over your chest, with palms facing and elbows slightly bent. Slowly lower by bending the elbows and spreading arms out in an arc fashion, as in Figure 1. Return to your starting position. Inhale as you lower, exhale on the lift. Lift for a count of 1, lower for a count of 2. Always resist the weight as you lower it.

Figure 2 - Chest Press. (This exercise works the major muscles of the chest, shoulders and triceps.) With palms facing forward, hold the weights side by side to your shoulders, as in Figure 2. Press weights towards the ceiling for a full extension without locking the elbows. Return to start position. Exhale as you press the weights upwards. Inhale as you lower.

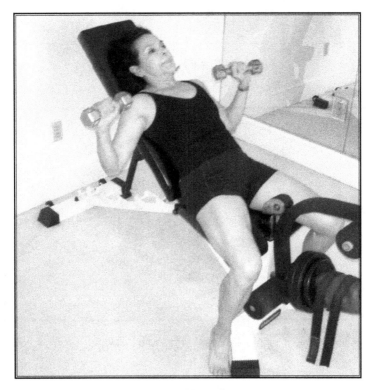

Figure 2 - Chest Press

Figures 3 & 4 - Flyes and Press. In lieu of a bench, pillows work very well, as you can see in Figures 3 and 4. When the chest, shoulders and head are elevated, the pec muscle can be worked more efficiently for faster results.

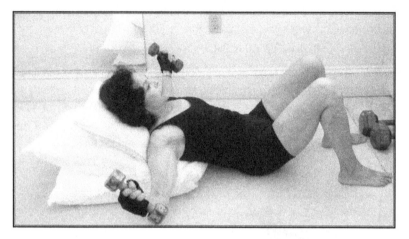

Figure 3 - Chest Flye with Pillow

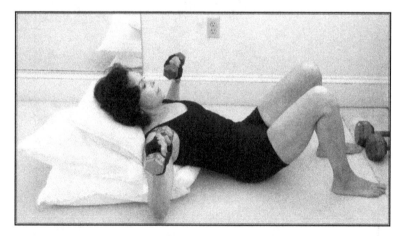

Figure 4 - Chest Press with Pillow

SHOULDER EXERCISES
(middle, anterior, posterior deltoid)

Shoulder exercises strengthen the deltoid muscle. It sits over the shoulder joint and is involved in every lifting move we make while protecting the shoulder joint from injury.

Figure 1 - Shoulder Press. (This exercise strengthens the middle shoulder.) Hold the weights side by side to your shoulders, palms facing forward. Press the weight towards the ceiling for a full extension without locking the elbows. Return to your starting position and repeat. Exhale on lift, inhale as you lower.

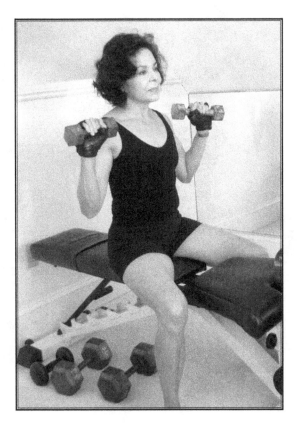

Figure 1- Shoulder Press

Figure 2 - Shoulder Front Lift. (This exercise strengthens the posterior shoulder.) Begin with the weights by your side, palms facing inward. Lift the arm as a unit, with elbows slightly bent until weights are even with your shoulders. Return to your starting position and repeat. Exhale on the lift, inhale as you lower.

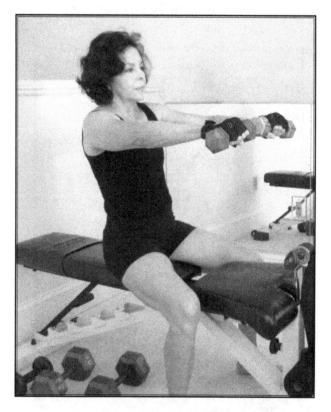

Figure 2 - Shoulder Front Lift

Figure 3 - Side Lateral. (This exercise strengthens the middle shoulder.) Start with arms at a 45-degree angle, pressed to your sides. Lift the arms as a unit from the shoulder until elbows, shoulders and weights are on an even plane. Return to your starting position. Repeat. Exhale on the lift.

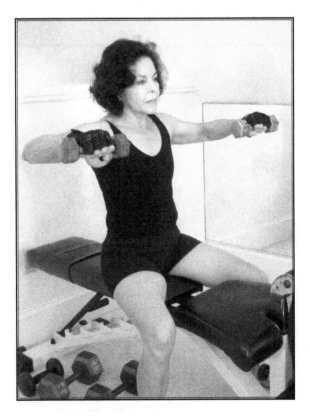

Figure 3 - Shoulder Side Lateral

Figure 4 - Rear Deltoid. (This exercise strengthens the rear shoulder.) Sit with knees together. Keeping your back flat (not rounded) slowly lower your chest as close to your quads as you can. Hold the weights over your feet, with palms facing each other. Bend the elbows slightly and holding the arms as a unit, push up with the upper arms towards the ceiling. Slowly lower and repeat. Lift for a count of 1, lower for a count of 2. Always resist the weight as you lower it.

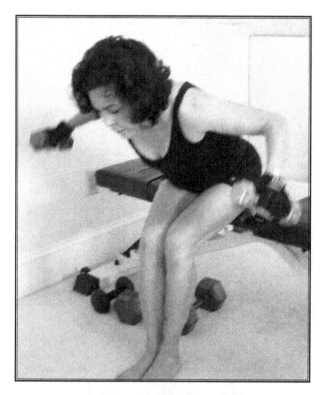

Figure 4 - Shoulder Rear Deltoid

ARMS & BACK EXERCISES
(biceps, triceps, lats)

The biceps muscle is used in flexion (push/pull) of the arm. The triceps muscle is involved in extension of the elbow and forearm. The lat muscles stabilize the torso and provide force in a variety of body positions.

Figure 1 - Biceps Curl. (This exercise strengthens the front of the arm.) Start with your arms down at your sides, holding the weights with palms facing forward, and elbows slightly bent. Press the weights upward and contract the biceps muscles. Keep your upper arms steady and at your sides. Slowly lower and repeat. Resist as you lower the weight. Exhale on the lift.

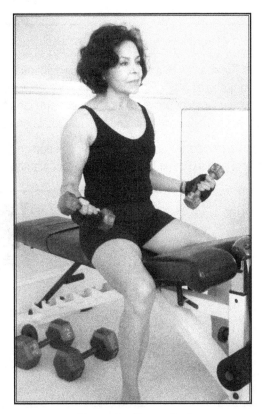

Figure 1 - Biceps Curl

Figure 2 - Lying Triceps. (This exercise strengthens the backs of the arms). Lie on your back with knees bent. Start with the arms at a 45-degree angle, palms facing inward. Lift for a full extension without locking the elbows. Lower and repeat. Exhale on the lift.

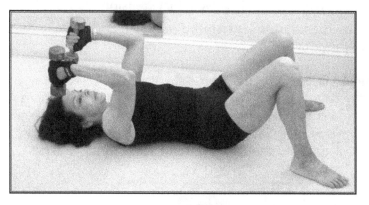

Figure 2 - Lying Triceps

Figure 3 - Triceps Kickback. (This exercise also strengthens the backs of the arms.) Start with your arm at a 45-degree angle, elbow slightly higher than your back and pressed to your side. Slowly straighten your arm for a full extension without locking the elbow. Slowly lower and repeat. Exhale on the extension.

This exercise can also be done on a bench with one knee on the pad, back parallel to the floor and the other leg straight with foot planted on the floor.

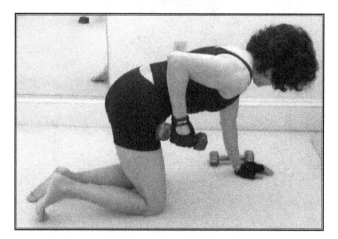

Figure 3 - Triceps Kickback

Figure 4 - Back Row. (This exercise strengthens the mid-back muscles). Sit with knees together. Keeping your back flat, lower your torso as close to your legs as possible. Start with arms at your sides, palms facing inward, weights by your ankles. Bend the arm at the elbow and push with your upper arm towards the ceiling as far as you can. Exhale as you lift. Resist as you lower the weight.

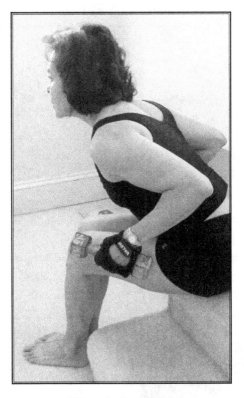

Figure 4 - Back Row

ABDOMINAL EXERCISES

(rectus abdominis, obliques)

The abdominal muscles support the trunk and provide postural and spinal support.

Figure 1 - Pelvic Tilt. (This exercise strengthens the pelvis and abdominals.) Lie on your back with knees bent, feet shoulder-width apart. Keeping your lower back pressed into the floor, lift the pelvis towards your navel, contracting the abdominal muscle. Hold for one second, and lower. Repeat. Exhale on the contraction or the lift.

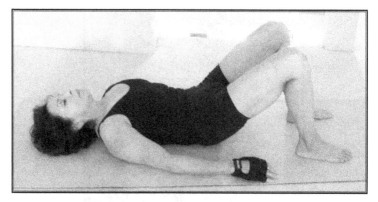

Figure 1 - Pelvic Tilt

Figure 2 - Hip Raise. (This exercise strengthens the hip area.) The alignment for the Hip Raise is the same as for the Pelvic Tilt. Raise your hips and consciously contract the abdominal muscle as you lift. Hold and exhale. Repeat.

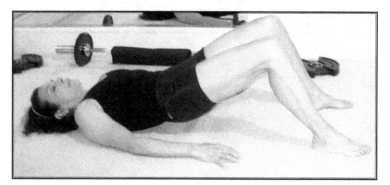

Figure 2 - Hip Raise

Figures 3 & 4 - Balanced & Modified Knees to Chest. (This exercise is both an abdominal strengthener and a balancing move.) If you have difficulty balancing yourself, start with Figure 4, with hands on the floor for support. With experience you'll be able to balance yourself without holding on to the floor.

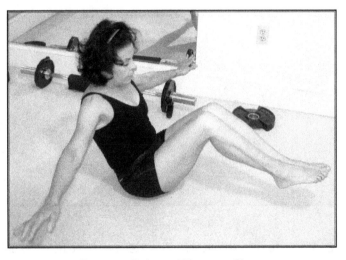

Figure 3 - Balanced Knees to Chest

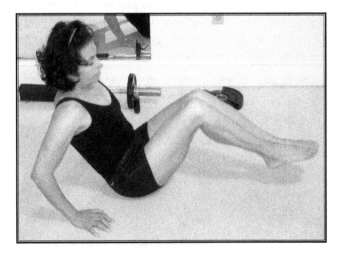

Figure 4 - Modified Knees to Chest

Figure 5 - Crunch. (This exercise strengthens the abdominal muscles.) Lie flat on your back with knees bent and out to the side. (This is important because if your knees are together, you will be using your hip flexor muscles instead of your abdominals.) Slowly raise your head and shoulders off the floor keeping them together as a unit. Curl your shoulders forward as if rolling a piece of paper. You will face your legs. At the top of the movement, contract your abdominal muscles and slowly lower to your starting position. If you have a problem with your neck, use one hand for support.

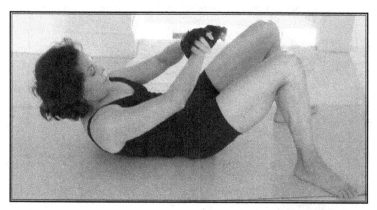

Figure 5 - Crunch

Figure 6 - Elbow to Opposite Knee. (This exercise strengthens the oblique muscles.) (Use the same starting alignment as Figure 5.) Lift your right leg and hold at a 45-degree angle, while placing your left foot on top of your right knee. Place your right hand behind your head for support and hold your left arm straight out. Press right shoulder to left knee. Exhale as you contract the abdominal muscle. Do as many reps as you can, then switch.

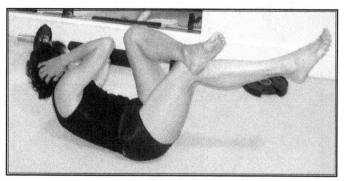

Figure 6 - Elbow to Opposite Knee

GLUTES & LEG EXERCISES

(gluteus maximus, quadriceps, hamstrings, gastrocnemius, inner thigh)

Glutes and leg exercises strengthen and tone the butt and the leg muscles from all four sides.

Figure 1 - Dead lift. (This exercise strengthens the glutes and lower back.) Stand with your legs straight or slightly bent. Hold weights or barbell in front of your legs. Keeping your back flat, slowly bend at the hips, without rounding your back. Return to an upright position and repeat. Inhale as you lower the weight, exhale as you lift.

Warning: Skip this exercise if you have back or knee problems.

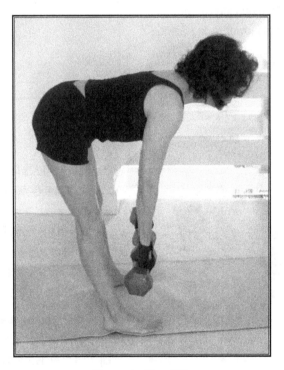

Figure 1 - Dead lift

Figure 2 - Calf Raise. (This exercise stretches and tones the calf muscle.) Stand on the edge of a step holding on to a railing and position your feet so you are standing on the balls of your feet. Go up on your toes as much as comfortable then contract the calf muscle. Slowly lower your heels to stretch the calf muscle. Repeat. Exhale on the contraction or lift.

Figure 3 - Squat. (The squat tones the glutes [butt] and legs as well as strengthens the lower back.) Stand

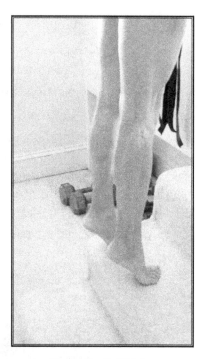

Figure 2 - Calf Raise

with your feet shoulder-width apart and toes pointed slightly outward. Lower your quads and butt until you are parallel to the floor. Return to an upright position without locking your knees. Repeat. Inhale as you lower, exhale on the lift.

Warning: If you have any kind of knee, lower back or ankle problem, skip this exercise. Instead, work your glutes by doing the Glute Press shown on page 85.

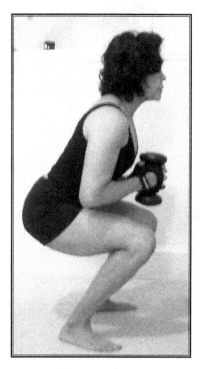

Figure 3 - Squat

Figure 4 - Hamstring Curl. (This exercise strengthens the hamstring muscle.) Lie on a bench face down. Place your ankles under the roller and lift until your heels are above your knee. Keep your back flat, do not overarch. Slowly lower the weight without locking your knees.

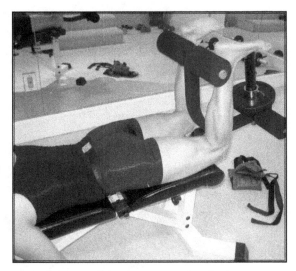

Figure 4 - Hamstring Curl

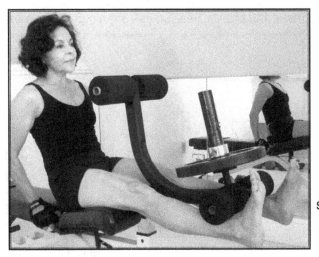

Figure 5 - Quadriceps Extension

Figure 5 - Quadriceps Extension. (This exercise strengthens the quad muscle.) Place your instep behind the roller and lift until the legs are almost straight. Lower with control. Repeat. Exhale on the lift.

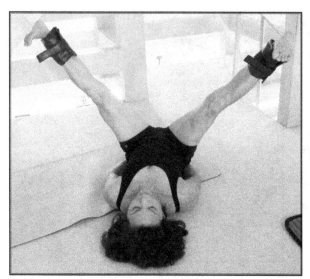

Figure 6 - Inner Thigh. (This exercise strengthens the inner thigh muscle.) Lie on your back with your hands under your rear. Bring your knees into your chest and straighten your legs upward keeping them straight. Slowly open your legs being careful not to overstretch. Repeat.

Figure 6 - Inner Thigh

Figure 7 - Outer Thigh. (Best exercise for outer thigh bulges.) Position yourself as you see in the picture, legs at a 45-degree angle. Lift your whole leg as a unit until parallel to the hip. Lower and repeat. Do as many repetitions as you can. Your goal is to get to 40-50. This may sound like a lot of repetitions, but to tone and tighten your thigh, high repetitions are necessary. It takes a lot of work to burn the fat stored in the thigh.

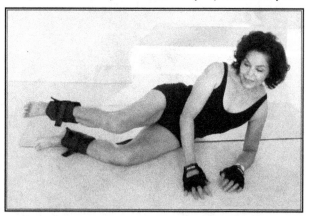

Figure 7 - Outer Thigh

When you can complete 40 to 50 reps and are ready to use an ankle weight, start with 5 pounds on each ankle. Build up to 40 to 50 reps. When you can do this with ease, increase the weight and place it on top of your thigh. Work your way up to 40 to 50 reps again. Take breaks and stretch by bringing the knee into the chest when you need to, then keep going. Sometimes called the hydrant, this exercise leans your thighs better than any machine available.

Alternate Legs

Alternate-leg exercises offer you another choice to leg training. If you don't have a bench with a leg attachment to work quads and hamstrings, or you are unable to perform squats for physical reasons, you can do the exercises provided using ankle weights.

Figure 1 - Glute Press with ankle weight. (This is an excellent exercise to tone the rear-end if you cannot do squats. I have seen women reduce their bottoms to an amazing degree by doing Glute Presses with ankle weights. You just have to do enough of them!) If you have a problem resting on your wrists, you can bend the arm and rest on your elbows. Begin with knees together hip-width apart. Flex your left foot and bend the leg to a 45 degree angle. Lift the whole leg as a unit until your knee is nearly parallel to the hip. Keep abs tucked in tight and your back flat.

Before you begin using an ankle weight, be sure your alignment is correct. I start beginners without a weight. Once they can do 40 repetitions on each leg, then they move on to the weights.

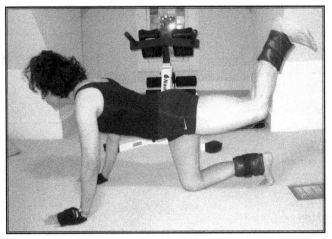

Figure 1 - Glute Press with ankle weight

Figure 2 - Hamstring Curl with ankle weight. This is one way of working your hamstrings even if you do not have a bench with a foot attachment. For this exercise, you can start using the ankle weights from the beginning. Begin with your legs together, straight out on the floor. Flex your feet and lift both legs until your ankles are over your knees. Consciously contract the hamstring muscle. Exhale as you lift. Lower and repeat.

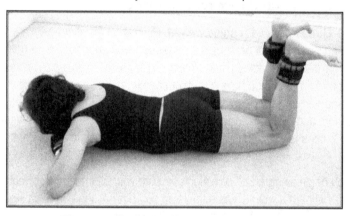

Figure 2 - Hamstring Curl with ankle weight

Figure 3 - Quad Extension with ankle weight. (This exercise strengthens the quad muscle.) Sit with your chest up and abdominals tight. Strap on an ankle weight and lift your lower leg until it's almost straight. Do not lock the knee. Lower and repeat. Exhale on the lift.

Figure 3 - Quad Extension with ankle weight

STRETCHING EXERCISES

These stretches can be performed before, during or after your exercise routine. Stretch lightly before your routine just to get your blood flow going. During your routine, another quick stretch will keep your muscles loose. After your routine, when your muscles are warmed up, you can spend more time stretching your muscles, challenging them a bit more.

Hold all stretches for a count of 20. Breathe and relax into the stretch. Concentrate on the word "relax".

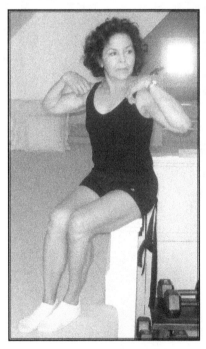

Figure 1 - Shoulder stretch. With hands on your shoulders, make a circle with your elbows. 10 forward, 10 back.

Figure 2 - Chest stretch. Clasp hands behind your back. Press down while raising your ribcage.

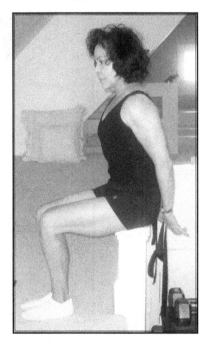

Figure 1 - Shoulder Stretch

Figure 2 - Chest Stretch

Figure 3 - Back stretch. Extend your arms in front of you. Clasp your hands and round your back like a bow.

Figure 4 - Calf stretch. Stand on the edge of a step while holding on to a railing or ledge. Place your feet so you can rest on the balls of your feet with the heels fully stretched downward. Bend one knee and hold the stretch on the opposite foot. Count to 20. Move slowly through this stretch. Switch legs. Stretch one, relax the other.

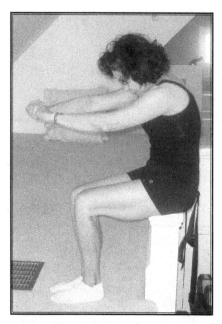

Figure 3 - Back Stretch

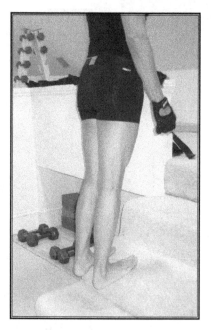

Figure 4 - Calf Stretch

Figure 5 - Quadriceps stretch. Stand with your feet shoulder-width apart. Hold on to a chair. Reach down and grab one ankle. If this is difficult, use a strap. Keeping your quad steady, lift your ankle towards your hamstring. Hold and breathe. Do not force the stretch. Keep knees side by side, torso lifted chest high and abs in.

Figure 6 - Lower-back stretch. Lie flat on your back with knees bent. Lift your knees towards your chest and slowly drop them to one side. If you cannot lower them to the floor, only lower as much as you can. Switch and roll legs to the other side.

Warning: If you have lower-back problems, skip this stretch or do it only after you have checked with your doctor.

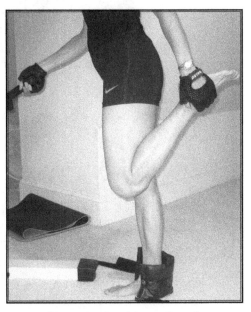

Figure 5 - Quadriceps Stretch

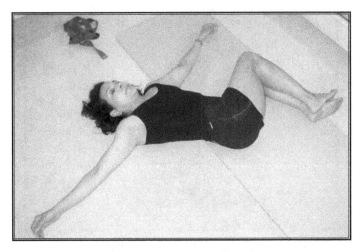

Figure 6 - Lower-back Stretch

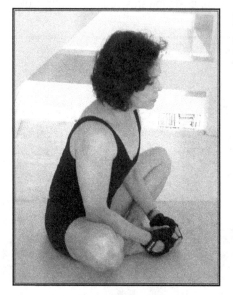

Figure 7 - Inner Thigh Stretch

Figure 7 - Inner-thigh stretch. Sit with soles of your feet facing each other. Lift your chest and press abdominals in. Lean forward as much as you can and press your knees to the floor. You can also reach with your arms and walk your hands away from your feet. Hold and breathe.

Figure 8 - Hamstring stretch. Lie flat on your back. If you have a hard time reaching your leg, use a yoga strap or towel. Lift one leg while keeping the other one bent. Flex your foot and slowly bring your leg towards your chest.

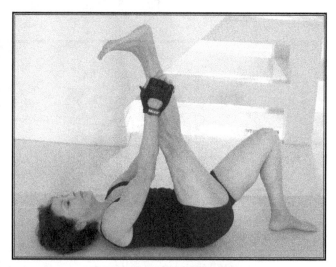

Figure 8 - Hamstring Stretch

MY WORKOUT, MYSELF

My training goal has always been to be as strong as possible. I always challenge myself to lift as much weight as I can. I am not worried about bulking up, in fact, even after 25 years of training I would still like to have more muscle than I do!

Figure 1: Here I am doing bicep curls with 25-pound dumbbells. I start out with 20 pounds and then do my last set of 10 with 25 pounds.

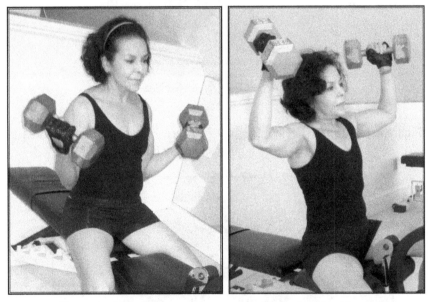

Figure 1 - Biceps Curl   Figure 2 - Shoulder Press

Figure 2: Shoulder presses with 25-pound dumbbells take my breath away, but I love that I can do this! Building a strong trunk (shoulders, core and hips) has made my quest for proper posture possible.

Figure 3: On a regular chest workout day, I do 35 repetitions of chest flyes with 35-pound dumbbells, in addition to the usual presses and pullovers.

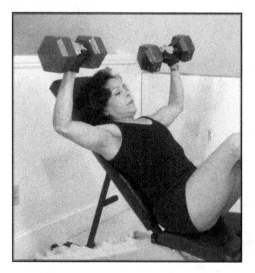

Figure 3 - Chest Press & Flyes

Figure 4: My favorite stretch is the plow. Though it took years to master, I was determined to do it—a great stretch for the lower back.

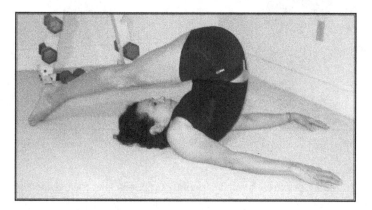

Figure 4 - Lower Back Plow

Figure 5: When I began this stretch 20 years ago, I could only reach my knees. Little by little I reached further and further down my legs with the goal of touching my forehead to my knees. I was thrilled when I could finally do it!

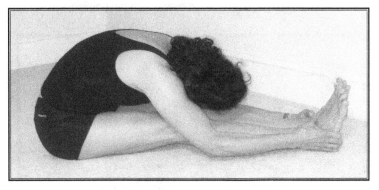

Figure 5 - Stretch

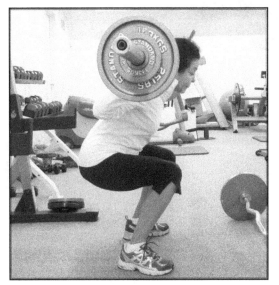

Figure 6 - Squat

Figure 6: Here I am squatting with a 100-pound barbell. On this particular day I could do 10 reps after I had warmed up with 90, then 95 pounds—my 69th birthday present to myself and again on my 70th birthday. Squatting is my passion! I plan to be squatting when I'm 100 years old!

As you may remember from the introduction, before I began training I had been diagnosed with a deteriorating spine that would eventually need surgery. Squats and dead lifts healed and strengthened my spine, so today I feel I can do anything!

Figure 7: I love this chest-pullover exercise and most everyone else I have taught does too! Here I am training with a 40-pound dumbbell. I can do two sets of 15 reps. Chest pullovers have helped me heal my nagging shoulder problem that had become chronic before I began training.

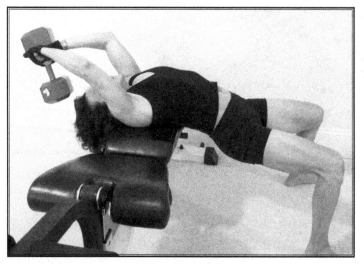

Figure 7 - Pullover

CHAPTER SIX
Nutrition: You Are What You Eat

"People who ate the most animal-based foods got the most chronic disease. Even relatively small intakes of animal-based foods were associated with adverse effects. People who ate the most plant-based foods were the healthiest and tended to avoid chronic disease." [1]

—T. Colin Campbell, Ph.D. and Thomas M. Campbell II

(Dr. T. Colin Campbell has been at the forefront of nutrition research for more than 40 years. His legacy, *The China Study*, is the most comprehensive study of health and nutrition ever conducted.)

In my 25-year search for healthy nutrition information, I have reviewed hundreds of scientific studies on diets most likely to lower the risk of developing degenerative diseases and promote health and vitality throughout life. Nearly every study points to a plant-based diet.

The longest living people in the world eat a vegetarian diet. They experience the fewest incidences of heart disease, cancer,

---

[1] Campbell, T. Colin, Ph.D. with Campbell, Thomas M. III, *The China Study, Startling Implications for Diet, Weight Loss and Long-Term Health* (Dallas: BenBella Books, Inc., 2006) p. 7.

diabetes, osteoporosis and Alzheimer's—the diseases that kill millions of Americans every year. They consume lots of fresh fruits, vegetables, grains, nuts and seeds with an occasional glass of wine. They find their primary source of protein through legumes, grains, yogurt and cheese. Olive oil is their principal source of fat.

THE ORNISH DIET

Dr. Dean Ornish, founder of the Preventive Medicine Research Institute in Sausalito, California, was the first clinician to demonstrate that a comprehensive program of lifestyle changes could both prevent and reverse heart disease. The Ornish Diet, also known as The Life Choice Diet, is a vegetarian diet.[2]

The diet calls for a ratio of 10 percent fat (15 to 25 grams of fat per day), 15-20 percent protein, and 70-75 percent complex carbohydrates. Dr. Ornish's recommendations contrast dramatically with the typical American diet, which features 40 percent fat, 20 percent protein and 40 percent carbohydrates.[3]

The Ornish Diet focuses on fruits, vegetables, whole grains and legumes, while suggesting that individuals can eat as much of these foods as they need in order to satisfy their hunger. Dr. Ornish recommends mindful eating to prevent overeating. He also advises eating while sitting down at the dinner table, not standing or watching television. Eating smaller bites, smaller portions and focusing on the food's texture, all help to promote satiety without eating more than a given body needs.[4]

In the Ornish Diet, foods to avoid include all meats, including chicken and fish, as well as oils, sugar, full-fat dairy products and alcohol. When an individual eliminates these foods, says

---

[2] http://www.dietsinreview.com/diets/Ornish_Diet/
[3] http://fatfree.com/diets/ornish.html
[4] http://diet.lovetoknow.com/wiki/Dean_Ornish_Diet

Dr. Ornish, counting fat grams or calories, becomes unnecessary. The health impact of this diet can be dramatic. As a result of their new diets and other lifestyle changes, Dr. Ornish's heart disease patients not only reversed their coronary artery blockages, but also gained energy and lost weight.

Weight loss is due in part to a plant-based diet that promotes a feeling of fullness. Though deviating from the Ornish protocol, in its inclusion of chicken and fish, a study at the University of Alabama revealed that when allowed to eat as much as they wanted of high-quality, wholesome foods—fruits, vegetables, soups, salads, fish, chicken and brown rice—people felt satisfied with as few as 1,500 calories per day. By contrast, those who consumed refined, processed foods—bacon, eggs, juice, buttered toast, steak, cake, ice cream and fast foods of all kinds—needed 3,000 calories to feel satisfied.

THE CHINA PROJECT

The China Project, a massive study to examine the relationship between diet, lifestyle and disease-related mortality, followed 6,500 Chinese people from 1983 to 1990. A joint project of Cornell University, Oxford University and Chinese scientists, the study focused primarily on the diets and lifestyle of rural Chinese people.[5]

The rural Chinese diet is mainly plant-based. The study showed that nutrients usually present in plant-based foods do minimize the occurrence of chronic degenerative diseases. The risk of chronic disease and elevated cholesterol increased when animal foods were introduced to an existing plant-based diet.

---

[5] Campbell, T. Colin, Ph.D. with Campbell, Thomas M. III, Lyman, Howard, and Robbins, John. *The China Study: The Most Comprehensive Study of Nutrition Ever Conducted and the Startling Implications for Diet, Weight Loss and Long-Term Health* (Dallas: BenBella Books, Inc., 2006)

The chart below shows the difference between the typical, rural Chinese diet and the typical American diet: [6]

Nutrient	China	U. S.
Calories	2641	1989
Total fat (% of calories)	14.5	34-38
Dietary fiber (g/day)	33	12
Total protein (g/day)	64	91
Animal protein (% of calories)	0.8	10-11
Total iron (mg/day)	34	18

As you can see, the Chinese consume, on average, 600 more calories than Americans, yet they eat a third less fat, three times the fiber, a third less protein (with animal protein at less than 1 percent) and double the iron than the average American.

Even though the rural Chinese consume 30 percent more calories than Americans, they weigh, on average, 20 percent less and have virtually no overweight problems. Why do we tend to be so much heavier, when we consume fewer calories? Eating a high-fat, high-protein diet (typical American fare) causes the body to retain more calories than it needs. The body then stores these extra calories as body fat. Retaining only 50 extra calories per day can create an extra 10 pounds of weight gain per year. Over a period of five years, that's a 50-pound gain!

The China Project provided further proof that a plant-based diet is far healthier than an animal-based one. Called the "Grand Prix of Epidemiology" by *The New York Times,* the China Project

---

[6] Ibid, p. 74

has produced more than 8,000 statistically significant associations between different dietary factors and disease. "We are basically a vegetarian species," concludes T. Colin Campbell, Ph.D., one of the lead researchers. "We should be eating a wide variety of plant foods and minimizing our intake of animal foods."

Dr. Campbell, at the forefront of nutritional research for more than 40 years, described his 20-year journey with this project in a book entitled *The China Study: The Most Comprehensive Study of Nutrition Ever Conducted and the Startling Implications for Diet, Weight Loss and Long-Term Health* [7]. Some of Dr. Campbell's findings follow:

Chronic Disease. People who ate the most animal-based foods suffered the most chronic disease. People who ate the most plant-based foods were the healthiest and inclined toward avoiding chronic disease.[8]

Osteoporosis. Animal protein decreases bone health. Animal protein promotes acid in the process of metabolism and leaches calcium from the bones. A 1993 report on protein intake and fracture rates issued by researchers at Yale University School of Medicine found that 70 percent of the fracture rate for women in the study was attributable to the consumption of animal protein. Even though Americans consume more milk and milk products per person than most countries in the world (for supposed personal-health reasons); American women, age 50 and older, have one of the highest rates of fractures in the world.[9]

Eye Problems.[10] At least 70-88 percent of blindness caused by macular degeneration—the leading cause of blindness among

---

[7] Ibid
[8] Ibid, p. 7
[9] Ibid, p. 204-205
[10] Ibid, p. 215-217

people over 65—can be prevented by a healthy diet. Researchers have found that people who eat a diet high in carotenoid antioxidants have lower incidence of macular degeneration. Green leafy vegetables, carrots and citrus fruits provide an important source of these nutrients.

In 2006, Dr. Campbell said that after 20 years of research, the China Project changed not only the way he thought about nutrition and health, but also the way he and his family eat. He stopped eating almost all animal-based foods, including meat and dairy, except on very rare occasions. His wife Karen created an entirely new dietary lifestyle for the entire family. The result is that he's more physically fit now than when he was 25, and is now at an ideal weight for his height.

He added that, "There are virtually no nutrients in animal-based foods that are not better provided by plants." [11]

YOU ARE WHAT YOU EAT

Learning about healthy nutrition is a duty we owe ourselves. Food makes us who we are. The foods we eat nourish our hair, skin, nails, organs, tissues, ligaments, tendons and nerves. Our nutritional intake affects our ability to think, process information, express our self, hold down a job and maintain healthy relationships with our loved ones. Food affects how we feel, and therefore how we relate to everyone and everything around us. It also affects our posture, our ability to stretch and move easily and our body image.

Considering that nutritional value affects not only how we look but also how we feel will help us make healthy food choices. When we give our body good nutrition, it will reflect our vigor and vitality.

---

[11] Ibid, p. 230

I did not learn about nutrition from the latest fad diet on the best-seller list. I went to the scientists who were doing the research. They inspired me to change my diet. I make conscious nutritional choices that boost my immune system, prevent illness and develop the strength and vigor I need to live, train and stretch my potential well beyond my 70s, 80s and 90s.

I can only recommend what I practice, thus my primary nutritional recommendation is simple: eat a plant-based diet.

A plant-based diet concerns some athletes, as they wonder where they will get their protein. The old notion that a complete protein combines plant-based foods such as rice and beans no longer holds true. Dr. Campbell explains that by eating a vegetarian diet rich in a broad range of vegetables over the course of a day can provide the body with all of the essential amino acids it needs for muscle growth and repair.

My basic nutritional program consists of the following food groups and simple rules:

FOOD GROUPS

Fat - Healthy fats include olive oil, Omega-3 fatty acids, fish oil, nuts and seeds. The typical American diet consists of 40 to 50 percent fat. Reducing fat intake to promote good health can begin by eating a vegetarian meal once or twice a week. This will cut fat, increase fiber, foster weight loss and increase energy.

Protein - Healthy sources of protein include vegetables, legumes (beans, lentils and peas), quinoa pasta or grain (13 grams of protein per 3.5 oz. serving), soy products, fish and yogurt.

Carbohydrates - Healthy complex carbohydrates high in fiber include: fruits, vegetables and whole grains (brown rice, buckwheat, barley and bulgur). Unhealthy simple carbohydrates low in fiber include: sweets, white bread, white rice, white potatoes and white pasta.

SIMPLE RULES TO FOLLOW:

- ✓ Eat a plant-based diet consisting of vegetables, fruits, whole grains, nuts and seeds.
- ✓ Eat fish twice weekly, including salmon at least once.
- ✓ Eat fruits low in sugar, such as berries, melons, oranges, apples and pears.
- ✓ Whenever possible, eat organic produce, locally grown and in season. Locally grown, fresh, seasonal ingredients retain their flavor and nutritional value because they have not been stored in warehouses for extended periods of time. The shorter the time from farm to table, the healthier, and the less need to enhance flavor.
- ✓ Eat only until 80% full.
- ✓ For protein, eat fish and legumes, soy products, grains and nuts.
- ✓ Use olive oil for cooking and salad dressings.
- ✓ Flavor foods with healing spices (cinnamon, cayenne, bay leaf, oregano) and herbs (garlic, ginger, fennel, red pepper).
- ✓ Drink tea 2 to 3 times per day.
- ✓ Use cheese sparingly, for flavoring, not as a staple. Choose cheeses like Italian Parmigiano-Reggiano and Spanish Pata Cabra goat cheese. Both these cheeses have a strong, sharp taste. A little goes a long way.
- ✓ Avoid fruit juices (very high sugar content) and instead eat fruit or drink filtered water.
- ✓ Eat small meals of about 300 calories, five times per day. Our body burns this small amount of calories and has nothing left to store as fat.

✓ Drink eight glasses of water daily.

✓ Use cayenne pepper to enhance flavors. Cayenne pepper is used worldwide to treat a variety of health problems, such as poor circulation, poor digestion, chronic pain, sore throat and gas. Cayenne pepper contains Vitamin C, E and carotenoids.

✓ Avoid eating foods cooked at high-temperatures as the charred and grilled-marked surfaces can contain carcinogens.

COOKING METHODS

Cooking methods to enhance flavor and cut fat are: baking, braising, broiling, poaching, roasting, sautéing and stir-frying. All these cooking methods require little or no fat. Substitutes for fat can be marinades made of citrus, such as orange, lemon and grapefruit juices, soy sauce, mirin (Asian sweet rice wine), tomato sauce, fat-free chicken/vegetable broth, herbs and spices.

Notice that I have not included grilling in my list of recommended cooking methods. Even though many consider grilling to be healthy, there has long been a connection between grilling and carcinogens.

I stopped eating grilled foods more than 20 years ago when I read that charring and smoking food at high temperatures create toxic compounds linked to cancer and other diseases. I cringe when I watch a cooking show and the chef or cook salivates over "the smoky flavor of grill marks."

According to The Cancer Project, a program of The Physicians Committee for Responsible Medicine,[12] grilling can be healthy if the food you grill is *not meat, chicken, pork, salmon or*

---

[12] http://www.cancerproject.org/media/news/fiveworstfoodsreport.php

hamburgers. According to The Cancer Project, all of these foods can produce the highest levels of cancer-causing compounds called heterocyclic amines (HCAs), when grilled at high heat for long periods of time. HCAs form when creatine (an amino acid found in muscle) and sugars, both found in meats, are heated during cooking. HCAs can bind directly to DNA, cause mutation, and promote the beginnings of cancer.

The Cancer Project is a collaborative effort of physicians, researchers and nutritionists who have joined together to educate the public about the benefits of a healthy diet for cancer prevention and survival.

In January of 2005, the federal government officially added HCAs to its list of known carcinogens.[13]

Unfortunately, grilling chicken and fish is equally as dangerous to our health, according to The Cancer Project report. In fact, chicken produces more than ten times the amount of the carcinogenic HCAs found in meat. Grilled fish also produces the formation of HCAs.

To avoid cancer risk, give up grilling animal products and instead grill soy based veggie burgers or Portobello mushrooms.

For many of us who came from meat-eating families, the idea of cooking fish can be daunting. We think fish smells "fishy," when in fact newly caught fresh fish has a very "fresh and clean" smell. And we consider cooking fish to be complicated, when it can be quite simple.

Let me share *my* very first fish recipe. Buy freshly caught skinned fish fillets. Wash and pat your fish dry, and set it aside. Take a pot with a lid and dab the bottom with a teaspoon of olive oil. When the oil is medium hot, place a few tomato slices,

---

[13] http://ntp.niehs.nih.gov/ntp/roc/toc11.html

onion slices and chopped garlic into the oil. Place the fish on top of the vegetables and season with salt and cayenne pepper. Cover and cook at low to medium heat. After two to three minutes, turn the fish over and cook the other side. And that's it! You now have a delicious, lean and quick fish dish.

I have learned that cooking healthy does not have to be complicated or difficult.

Cookbook authors and restaurant chefs use lots of sugar, salt, oil, butter, bacon, pork and other meat parts to add flavor to the dishes they cook. This makes them fatty, salty and unhealthy. Our meals can be lean, delicious and nutritious, without added fat or sugar. We certainly don't need thick sauces made with flour and butter or flavorings like bacon or pork. These clog our arteries and make us fat. Once our taste buds become used to the natural and fresh taste of fruits and vegetables, we don't miss the fatty additives.

Eat lean to feel better, maintain or lose weight and avoid feeling bloated or sluggish.

EATING BEHAVIORS

How you eat is as important as *what* you eat.

People who have lost weight and kept it off for five years or more have adopted similar habits that have proven to be powerful tools in the weight-loss battle. Those are: keeping a food diary, weighing once a week and enjoying the company of like-minded people for moral support.

Keeping a food diary can help you change unconscious choices into conscious ones and monitor your progress and goals. A food diary can be your own internal coach. But you must be ready to face yourself and accept responsibility by being totally honest in your entries. Each day, enter the following information:

✓ Everything you ate, including meals and snacks

✓ Everything you drank: coffee, sodas, water and fruit juices

✓ The times for each meal and snack

✓ Your feelings before and after eating

✓ Your hunger level before each meal

✓ Your exercise routine

All this information will reveal your habits and practices and clarify what you may have been hiding from yourself about your eating. For example, were you really hungry when you ate that snack just one hour after lunch? Was your last meal eaten too late at night and were you watching TV as you ate it? Did you run out of the house without eating breakfast and instead grab a donut because you overslept?

Unless we face our destructive eating habits by uncovering and acknowledging our feelings and emotions, we'll be loathe to change. Awareness is the first step towards change, and change is the first step towards transformation. Avoid eating when angry, sad or lonely. Emotional eating is a double whammy. It promotes weight-gain and increases self-loathing. The best way to deal with emotional issues that make us unhappy is to express what we're feeling.

Eating behaviors run in families. Before I changed my eating habits, I never ate breakfast because my stomach was still full from the large meal I had eaten the night before. This was an eating pattern I had learned as a child. Upon reflection, I realized that I had to reverse that pattern if I was going to lose and maintain my weight, have better digestion and more sound sleep.

What destructive eating behavior can you link to your family of origin? Did your family also eat large meals, lots of junk food and/or fast foods? If you have adopted unhealthy eating behaviors that have caused you to gain weight and compromise your health, reflecting on the origin of these behaviors can help you realize that as an adult, you are now in control and can transform any limiting behavior.

MY DIET, MYSELF

Plants replace meat.

As inspired by the Ornish Diet, I wanted to cut my fat intake to as close to 10 percent as possible, so my first dietary change was to give up red meat.

Even though I had eaten meat all of my life, I did not find it difficult to give up the red meat after learning about its negative effects through my nutrition research.

"The bacteria in meat are identical to those in manure and more numerous in some meats than in fresh manure. All meats become infected with manure germs in the process of slaughtering. The number of manure germs increases while in storage. Meat is teeming with putrefactive bacteria or colon germs."[14]

I could not dismiss such information in addition to the numerous studies linking high meat consumption with colon cancer. Plus having suffered from constipation for half of my life, I wanted a clean colon. After only a few days on my meatless diet, my digestive system began to function much more efficiently with regular bowel movements. What a delight to feel light and more energetic.

Now that meat was no longer the centerpiece of every meal, I focused on fruits, vegetables, whole grains, legumes and fish. Olive

---

[14] Robbins, Anthony. *Unlimited Power* (New York, Fawcett Columbine, 1986) p.184

oil replaced butter for cooking and salad dressings. My new treats became breads and muffins, but later I also let these go.

Fruits replace sugar.

I used to begin my day with a muffin and a cup of coffee—sometimes even two muffins—as one muffin would barely fill me up since I usually woke up hungry from eating a very light dinner the night before.

When I looked in the mirror while brushing my teeth, I began to notice puffiness above my cheeks. It felt like a water bubble when I pressed on it—worse on some days than others. The unsightly, watery bumps soon concerned me, since I couldn't figure out what was causing them.

Then one day I saw Dr. Nicholas Perricone, dermatologist and author of *The Wrinkle Cure* [15], featured on a PBS special. "Beautiful skin doesn't come in a bottle; it comes from the inside out," he said. "It's the consequence of a nutritious diet and exercise." He went on to say that wrinkling and sagging skin is not the inevitable consequence of aging, but the result of damage caused by insufficient exercise, lack of sleep, excessive alcohol consumption and insufficient Vitamin A, C and E in the body and too much fat and sugar.

As soon as I heard the word "sugar," I made the connection between the puffiness in my face and the sugar in my muffins and sweet breads.

As I began to pay attention, I noticed that the puffiness around my eyes usually appeared the day after I had indulged in my beloved muffins—loaded with fat and sugar—as rich as cake, buttery and very sweet. Now that I knew the truth, I had

---

[15] Perricone, Nicholas, M.D., *The Wrinkle Cure* (New York: Time Warner Group, 2000)

a choice: I could continue to eat all that sugar and fat and look puffy and old, or as I had done before with meat, find a substitute for sugar. Giving up my "muffin addiction" wasn't easy. But in time I weaned myself from my sugar cravings. I found that as I cut back on sugar, my tastebuds became more sensitive to the taste of sugar. I then needed less and less sugar to be satisfied. My motivation to cut back on sugar increased when I learned about other detrimental effects that sugar has on our bodies.

It turns out that not only can a high-sugar diet cause skin to become puffy, dull and wrinkled due to inflammation; sugar can also damage your collagen and elastin. These are the protein fibers that support your skin, keeping it firm and elastic. Within a few weeks of reducing my sugar intake, my skin began to look noticeably firmer, as the puffiness dissipated.

I invite you to experiment on yourself. Do not use any added sugar for a week, and see what happens. If you must have something sweet, eat a piece of fruit. Focus on the sweetness of the fruit and tell yourself that's all you need. You might be surprised at the results.

It is important to realize that sugar can cause more serious damage than skin problems. As we age, our bodies become less able to break down glucose in the bloodstream. A study published in *Scientific American*[16] in 2009 linked rising levels of blood sugar to impairment of mental function. Study author Scott Small, a neurologist at Columbia University, and other researchers used an MRI to look at the effects of elevated blood glucose in the hippocampus (a part of the brain that plays an important role in long-term memory) of 181 men and women aged 65 or older with no history of dementia.

---

[16] http://www.scientificamerican.com/article.cfm?id=an-end-to-senior-moments

Those with higher levels of blood glucose suffered impairment of a section of the hippocampus that regulates age-related cognition such as forgetfulness. In Alzheimer's disease, the hippocampus is one of the first regions of the brain to suffer damage, causing memory lapses and disorientation.

Psychiatrist Mony de Leon of New York University, also cited in the article, believes that our ability to retain information can be improved when glucose intolerance is corrected.

Today, if I want something sweet, I eat a piece of fruit. Or I treat myself to a small bowl of homemade applesauce. I started making my own when I couldn't find a sugar-free version that I liked at the grocery store. I've included my applesauce recipe in the recipe section later in this chapter. Try it: I predict that you'll find it to be so delicious, you'll never want store-bought again!

Goodbye to Alcohol.

Alcohol was the last of my old habits to go. Some of you may be thinking that I've gone off the deep end, because you've heard that a glass of wine is good for your health, especially heart health. But "good for you" is debatable, because alcohol can also raise the risk for many types of cancer. How can a substance be good for one part of you and life-threatening for another? (If you want to do something for your heart health, try exercise. It has no negative side effects and it's good for every part of you!)

Alcohol also contributes to aging skin. Alcohol causes small blood vessels in the skin to dilate, and over time these tiny vessels can suffer permanent damage. We've all known heavy drinkers who have permanently flushed faces caused by broken blood vessels just under the surface of the skin.

The brain is particularly vulnerable to the effects of alcohol.[17]

---

[17] http://kidshealth.org/teen/drug_alcohol/alcohol/alcohol.html

Alcohol slows brain activity by suppressing the nervous system, that is, the brain, spinal cord and the nerves originating from it. As a result, messages to the brain become blocked or distorted. Alcohol alters perception, judgment, emotions, movement and even vision and hearing.[18]

I know what it is to suffer slurred speech, confused thinking and impaired coordination and balance because of alcohol. There was a time in my life when drinking was a nightly affair—sweet German wines were my favorite. I needed at least two or three glasses at the end of the day to take the edge off and be able to sleep. But usually I would wake in the middle of the night with palpitations that should have scared me, but didn't.

The fact that I never drank water was particularly dangerous, as my dehydrated body had no way of diluting the alcohol. We now know that female drinkers reach higher blood-alcohol levels faster than men because they carry more fat and less water in their bodies and also have different digestive enzymes. However, women develop alcohol-related disorders such as brain damage, cirrhosis and cancers at lower levels of drinking than men.

Radical aging—my concept that you can erase half your age by how you live your life—sometimes calls for major changes. Reflect on your nutritional intake, especially your alcohol, sugar and meat consumption, and follow your body's call to good health.

---

[18] http://oregoncounseling.org/articlespapers/documents/etohbiofx.htm

RECIPES

These recipes come from my own recipe library. I turn to them when I cook. Delicious and lean, they require few ingredients and can be prepared in minutes. These recipes provide the basis for developing countless others by substituting ingredients. For example, black beans for navy beans, pears for apples, baby portabellas for shiitakes and cabbage for bok choy. My Tomato Sauce can be used in soups, rice, egg and bean dishes.

When I grocery shop, I fill my basket with my favorite "super foods," ingredients packed with nutrition that I want in my diet for the coming week. My favorite "super foods" are: garlic, onions, tomatoes, spinach, sweet potatoes, some type of bean, salmon, a grain (quinoa, brown rice, barley) berries, apples and pears.

The ingredients in the following recipes are packed with both nutrition and medicinal qualities. These foods can reduce inflammation, regulate metabolism, burn body fat, stabilize blood pressure, help protect against chronic diseases and regulate digestion.

GRAINS

Basmati Rice with Chanterelle Mushrooms

Ingredients:	Preparation:
1 teaspoon olive oil 1 teaspoon chopped garlic 1 cup basmati rice 1 cup water 1 cup vegetable broth ½ teaspoon whole cumin seeds 1/8 teaspoon cardamom seeds ¼ teaspoon fennel seeds ¼ cup chopped shallots 2 cups chopped chanterelles, stems removed (or mushroom of your choice) salt, cayenne pepper	Sauté shallots and garlic in olive oil until soft. Do not let brown. Add seeds and mushrooms and sauté for 2 minutes. Add rice and blend with pan ingredients. Add water and broth. Season with salt and cayenne. Simmer uncovered stirring often. Cooking time is about 15-20 minutes. If the rice tastes a bit gritty, cover and let the steam finish cooking the rice.

Comment: Mushrooms are a great alternative to meat due to their chewy, dense consistency. Once you begin to use them in recipes, you won't miss meat. The seeds in this recipe can be substituted for either your favorite seed or sesame, flaxseed or pumpkin seeds. Seeds are packed with protein and fiber. You can also substitute brown rice for basmati. (Brown rice may take a little longer to cook.)

* add flaxseed & chia mix

Navy Bean, Spinach and Brown Rice Pilaf 🐟

Ingredients:	Preparation:
1 teaspoon olive oil 4 cups fresh spinach 1 cup navy beans with cherry tomatoes (see recipe below) 1½ cups cooked brown rice	Sauté spinach in olive oil, only until wilted. Add navy beans and brown rice. Toss to blend. Taste for seasoning.

Comment: This recipe is an example of how you can mix and match these meals to create quick, healthy, delicious and wholesome fare.

Quinoa Pasta with Vegetables

Ingredients:	Preparation:
1 package quinoa linguine 1 tablespoon olive oil 2 tablespoons garlic, chopped ⅓ cup red onion, chopped 2 small zucchini, halved lengthwise, cubed 3 small very ripe tomatoes, cubed 3 cups shiitake mushrooms, stemmed and sliced 1 tablespoon mixed herbs (oregano, thyme, rosemary), chopped ¼ cup Parmigiano-Reggiano, grated salt, cayenne	Heat olive oil on low setting. Add garlic and onions. Sauté until soft. Do not let brown. Add tomatoes, zucchini and mushrooms. Combine all ingredients. Stir often for about 10 minutes. The vegetables are done when the tomatoes' juices are released and the mushrooms are cooked, but not mushy. Season and set aside. Cook quinoa linguine according to package directions (see comment). When *al dente* (cooked but not mushy), drain. Serve pasta topped with vegetables. Sprinkle with grated cheese and fresh herbs.

Comment: Pasta cooking directions recommend adding olive oil to the cooking water. However, I often cook quinoa pasta and never add olive oil. Save yourself a lot of fat calories by using a fork to untangle the linguine as it hits the boiling water instead of using extra oil.

LEGUMES (BEANS AND LENTILS) ✗

Navy Beans with Cherry Tomatoes

Ingredients:	Preparation:
1 tablespoon olive oil ¼ chopped garlic ½ cup chopped onions 1 cup cherry tomatoes, halved 1½ cup dried navy beans 1 quart vegetable broth 1½ teaspoon chopped fresh herbs (rosemary, thyme and oregano sea salt, cayenne pepper)	Sauté garlic, onions and tomatoes in the olive oil. Simmer at low heat until soft. Add the beans and vegetable broth. Season and cover. Cook until beans are tender but not mushy. Stir in the herbs. Beans should be spicy and delicious.

Comment: Beans are high in protein and fiber. I cook a bean dish once a week. I freeze half and use the rest in tacos, as a side dish with eggs or as an addition to a pilaf.

Lentils with Sweet Potatoes ✗

Ingredients:	Preparation:
1 tablespoon of olive oil 2 tablespoon garlic, chopped ½ cup onion, chopped 2 tablespoon curry powder 1½ cup lentils 3 cups vegetable broth 3 cups sweet potatoes, peeled and diced 1 tablespoon chopped herbs (optional) salt, cayenne	Sauté garlic and onions in olive oil until soft. Add curry powder and stir for a few minutes. Add lentils and broth, then stir to combine. Cover and simmer for 15 minutes. Add sweet potatoes, cover and continue cooking until lentils are soft, 15-20 minutes. Lentils should be left with some of the broth, not completely dry. Season with salt and cayenne. Sprinkle with herbs.

Comment: A blend of medicinally potent spices: turmeric, cardamom, chili, cumin and coriander, curry powder is good for your brain.

Azuki Beans

Ingredients:	Preparation:
1 teaspoon olive oil 2 tablespoon chopped garlic ½ cup chopped onions 1¼ cup azuki beans 2 cups vegetable broth ½ cup canned San Marzano Tomato Sauce (or one of your choice)	Sauté onions and garlic in olive oil at low heat for 8-10 minutes. Add beans, broth and tomato sauce. Cover and simmer until beans are tender. Serve as a stuffing for taco, over brown rice or stir fry with spinach sautéed with garlic. Season with salt and cayenne.

Comment: Azuki beans are loaded with antioxidants, have a nutty flavor and are easy to digest. Among the beans, azukis contain the least amount of fat and the highest amount of protein.

SOUPS

Shiitake Soup

Ingredients:	Preparation:
1 tablespoon olive oil 1 head garlic, cloves peeled, chopped 4 cups leeks, white parts only, chopped 1 large potato, peeled, chopped 1½ quarts vegetable broth 4 cups shiitake mushrooms, sliced, stems removed salt, cayenne	Sauté garlic and leeks in olive oil until soft, 5-10 minutes. Add potato and broth. Cover and cook until potato is soft. Season with salt and pepper. Allow to cool. Purée using immersion blender.* Add shiitake mushrooms. Simmer for another 10 minutes and season.

Comment: An immersion blender is a hand-held electric device that can be inserted directly into a pot or bowl to purée foods. It's inexpensive, convenient and much easier to clean than a regular blender.

This soup is a delicious vegetarian alternative to using a heavy *roux*—nothing more than flour and fat—for thickening soup without the calories or sacrificing taste. Omitting the potato makes a lighter version. Any vegetable can be substituted; the possibilities are endless. Also, baby portabellas or oyster mushrooms can be substituted for shiitakes.

Navy Bean Soup with Spinach

Ingredients:	Preparation:
1 cup drained azuki beans, soaked overnight 1 tablespoon olive oil ⅓ cup chopped onions ¼ chopped garlic 4 cups vegetable broth 2 ounces baby spinach 1 teaspoon chopped herbs salt, cayenne	In a soup pot, heat oil at low heat and sauté onions and garlic for 10 minutes until caramelized.* Add vegetable broth and drained beans. Season with salt and cayenne. Cook covered until tender, approximately 40-45 minutes. Add spinach leaves and cook for another 5 minutes until spinach is wilted. Season with salt. Sprinkle with herbs.

Comment: *Vegetables are caramelized when their juices have reduced and become concentrated, intensifying their flavor. Depending on your particular stove, it may take longer than 10 minutes for onions to caramelize. Also, the amount of vegetable broth can be increased according to your taste.

Roasted Tomato and Garlic Soup with Greens

To roast tomatoes:

Place five medium chopped tomatoes, 1 tablespoon chopped garlic, ½ chopped onion and 1 tablespoon of olive oil in a bowl and toss to combine. Season with salt and cayenne pepper. Roast uncovered in the oven at 350° for 1½ hours or until juices are caramelized.

To make the soup:

Ingredients:	Preparation:
Roasted tomatoes and garlic mixture 1 quart vegetable broth 3 large carrots, sliced 1 large onion, chopped 1 bunch watercress, stems removed ½ bunch parsley, stems removed 1 large bok choy, stem removed, sliced	Place all ingredients in large soup pot and simmer covered for one hour. When cool, purée with immersion blender. Add salt and cayenne, to taste

Comment: This soup is thick and satisfying. Soups are a great way to get lots of vegetables in your diet. In the winter when tomatoes are out of season and not as flavorful, roasting them in olive oil with garlic and onions adds flavor.

Lentil and Tomato Soup

Ingredients:	Preparation:
1 tablespoon olive oil	Heat olive oil. Add onions,
⅓ cup garlic, chopped	garlic and carrots. Cook at
1 medium onion, chopped	low heat for 10-15 minutes
2 small carrots, diced	until vegetables are soft.
5 medium ripe tomatoes, diced	Add tomatoes and cook for
2 quarts vegetable broth	another 10 minutes. Add
2 cups lentils	vegetable broth and lentils.
1 tablespoon chopped herbs	Season. Cook until lentils
salt, cayenne	are soft, about 30 minutes.
	When soup is cool,
	purée in a blender or use
	immersion blender. Taste
	for seasoning and sprinkle
	with herbs.

Comment: This soup is thick and satisfying, great in winter. However, if you are a soup lover like me, it's wonderful year-round. One or two cups of this soup will nourish your body and your soul.

LOW-HEAT STIR FRY

Note: Cooking foods at low-heat helps to preserve nutrients.

Spinach Taco with *Cabra* Cheese

Ingredients:	Preparation:
1 whole wheat tortilla	Heat tortilla on both sides.
1 teaspoon olive oil	Spread cheese in the center
3 cups fresh spinach	and set aside. Sauté spinach
2 ¼-inch thick slices of *Pata Cabra*	in olive oil until wilted,
cheese	one minute. Season. Spoon
salt, cayenne	spinach on tortilla and fold.

Comment: This recipe makes a great snack or mini-meal. The *Pata Cabra* cheese is very pungent, so a little goes a long way. If handy, add a tablespoon of beans or tomato sauce to the taco.

Spinach, Shiitake Mushrooms and Garlic

Ingredients:	Preparation:
2 teaspoons olive oil	Heat olive oil and add
1 tablespoon chopped garlic	garlic and mushrooms.
1 cup shiitake mushrooms,	Simmer at low heat for 5
stemmed and chopped	minutes. Do not let brown.
5 oz. fresh baby spinach	Add spinach and cook until
1 teaspoon low-sodium soy sauce	wilted.
sea salt, cayenne pepper	Dowse with soy sauce. Toss
	to combine. Season to taste.

Comment: Any vegetable can be substituted for the spinach in this recipe (bok choy, cabbage, broccoli, cauliflower, yellow and red peppers, zucchini and tomatoes.)

Veggie Hash

Ingredients:	Preparation:
1 medium sweet potato, peeled, finely diced	Heat olive oil in a nonstick pan. Add sweet potatoes, garlic and onions and cook, stirring often for about 10 minutes. Add red pepper and continue cooking at low heat for another 10 minutes. Add spinach and cook for another 5 minutes. Total cooking time is about 25 minutes. When sweet potatoes are soft, add fresh herbs and season with salt and cayenne.
1 tablespoon olive oil	
1 medium red bell pepper, diced	
½ cup red onion, diced	
1 tablespoon garlic, chopped	
1 tablespoon fresh herbs, chopped	
3 cups baby spinach	
2 large eggs	
salt, cayenne pepper	

Comment: This delicious dish can also be enjoyed over rice, beans, stuffed into a tortilla or eaten alone. You can also add a diced yellow pepper. Be creative, substitute any of my ingredients for those you prefer and begin your own collection of recipes.

SAUCES

Tomato Sauce

Ingredients:	Preparation:
1 tablespoon olive oil ½ medium onion, chopped ⅓ cup chopped garlic 6 medium-size ripe tomatoes, chopped 1 tablespoons fresh herbs 1 cup chopped basil grated Parmesan cheese salt, cayenne pepper	Sauté onions and garlic in olive oil until softened. Add tomatoes. Crush with a fork. Blend and season. Simmer sauce for 30 minutes uncovered. When cool, remove ⅓ of the sauce and purée in a blender, then stir into the rest of the soup. You can also use an immersion blender. Add fresh herbs and basil and other seasonings, as desired. Sauce should be spicy.

Comment: If the amount of garlic suggested above is too much for you, adjust it. I like lots of garlic and basil. This tomato sauce has countless uses: a tablespoon can be stirred into an egg omelet or add a cup to a bean dish or a ¼ cup to a rice dish. One half cup can also be enjoyed for a quick snack. An immersion blender makes for easy puréeing since you don't have to pour liquids into a blender and then back into a soup pot. The blender goes right into the pot and blends.

Roasted Tomato Sauce

Ingredients:	Preparation:
5 medium chopped tomatoes 1 tablespoon chopped garlic ½ chopped onion 1 tablespoon olive oil salt and cayenne pepper	Roast in oven uncovered at 350° for 1½ hours or until juices are caramelized. Remove from oven and purée in blender.

Comment: You can use any type of onion (white, yellow, red or green). You can also use any variety of tomatoes (cherry, creole, roma, etc.) You can also add red or yellow bell peppers.

FISH
Salmon in Parchment

Ingredients:	Preparation:
½ lb. wild salmon 1 sliced tomato 1 teaspoon chopped garlic ¼ cup thinly sliced onion 1 tablespoon chopped herbs: rosemary, oregano and thyme salt, cayenne	Preheat oven to 425°. Take a one foot square piece of parchment paper and place inside a baking pan. In the center place the tomato slices, garlic and onions. Sprinkle with rosemary, oregano and thyme. Place fish on top and season. Take both ends of the parchment paper, roll tight and seal the ends. Bake for 15 minutes or less depending on desired doneness. Allow to cool before removing fish.

Comment: Cooking any fish in parchment paper saves on cleaning. Just throw the paper away and rinse the pan. There's no splattering on your stove or fishy smell afterwards.

Marinated Tuna

Ingredients:	Preparation:
2 ½-lb. tuna steaks **Marinade:** 1 tablespoon olive oil ¼ cup low sodium soy sauce 1 tablespoon lemon juice 1 tablespoon chopped garlic 1 tablespoon chopped ginger	Place fish in bowl and marinate for 20 minutes. Remove fish from marinade, dry and sauté in olive oil. Five minutes on each side or longer for desired doneness.

Comment: You can substitute orange juice for lemon juice. Adjust garlic and ginger to your own taste.

Open Face Sandwiches
Tomato and Basil Sandwich

Ingredients:	Preparation:
Whole grain, freshly-baked bread Heirloom tomato Basil and baby spinach leaves *Pata Cabra* Goat cheese Pear vinegar	Cut a thick slice of the bread and place on a plate. Layer thin slice of cheese over the bread, basil and spinach leaves and tomato slices, thickly sliced. Drizzle a teaspoon of the vinegar over the tomato slices and season with salt and sprinkles of cayenne.

Comment: I love open-faced sandwiches in the summer when tomatoes are sweet and delicious and basil plentiful. Heirloom tomatoes are highly prized for their desirable characteristics: sweet, fleshy and vibrantly colored (purple, yellow, pink and red). One slice of this sandwich makes a great snack. Two slices is a full meal.

Egg Sandwich with Basil and Tomato

Ingredients:	Preparation:
Two eggs sautéed in a dab of olive oil Whole grain freshly-baked bread Heirloom tomato Basil and baby spinach leaves *Pata Cabra* Goat cheese Pear vinegar	Cut a thick slice of the bread and place on a plate. Layer one egg, thin slices of cheese, basil and spinach leaves and tomato slices, thickly sliced. Drizzle a teaspoon of the pear vinegar over the tomato slices and season with salt and sprinkles of cayenne.

FRUIT

Chunky Applesauce

Ingredients:	Preparation:
4 Fuji or Gala apples, unpeeled, diced 1 Granny Smith apple, unpeeled, diced 1 tbsp. cinnamon zest of 1½ oranges zest of 1 lemon juice of 1½ oranges juice of ½ lemon	In a large pot combine the orange and lemon zests, and the juices of both orange and lemon. Add apples. Sprinkle cinnamon and toss to coat. Cover and simmer for about 15 minutes turning often. Once the apples have released their juices remove the cover and continue cooking. When cooked, apples will be soft, not mushy, juices caramelized.

Comment. This recipe takes a little patience, but it's worth it. As shared earlier, I developed this recipe because I found the store-bought applesauces too sweet. Spoon some of this applesauce over a sugar-free biscuit. It tastes like a delicious slice of apple pie—without the sugar, lard and butter. You're saving calories and eating healthier and more delicious fare.

Braised Pears

Ingredients:	Preparation:
5 ripe pears, unpeeled, seeded zest of 1 orange juice of 1 orange ground flax seeds	Combine all ingredients. Simmer, uncovered until juices have caramelized. Spoon over yogurt for a delicious treat or serve over cooked oatmeal topped with ground flax seeds or a handful of walnuts.

Comment: The pears natural sugars satisfy your sweet tooth. I make this recipe when pears are in season and lower in cost. The pears can also be substituted for apples of your choice.

Oatmeal with Apples and Orange Zest

Ingredients:	Preparation:
⅓ cup quick oats	Combine first four ingredients
½ cup water	in a saucepan.
½ cup almond milk	Cook, stirring often, for 2-3
¼ apple, thinly sliced	minutes. Add cinnamon and
1 teaspoon orange zest	orange zest.
dash of cinnamon	Toss to combine.
5 walnut pieces	

Comment: This oatmeal is so delicious that it can be eaten for breakfast, snack or dessert.

Apple and Prune Bake

Ingredients:	Preparation:
4 Cameo apples, cored, diced	Preheat oven to 425°.
5 pitted prunes, chopped	Combine all ingredients in
½ orange, juiced	a mixing bowl. Toss well
½ lemon, juiced	to combine flavors. Pour
zest of one lemon	apple mixture into a 10-inch
zest of one orange	baking pan and place in
1 teaspoon cinnamon	oven uncovered. Bake for 30
	minutes, remove from oven
	and toss. Place back in the
	oven for another 30 minutes.

Comment: This apple dish is slightly sweeter than the Chunky Applesauce because of the added prunes. Serve over yogurt or oatmeal.

* * *

My recipes give you an idea of how I prepare foods and what I eat every day: fresh fruits and vegetables cooked simply but with full flavor using herbs and plenty of garlic and onions for seasoning. For me, cooking is a joy. It's not only relaxing but also one way I express self-love and self-care.

I eat about four small meals per day. For breakfast I usually have oatmeal and fruit; mid-morning I'll have a spinach taco and my noon meal is usually soup or a vegetable omelet. Mid-afternoon, my last meal, could be fish (4 ounces) with a vegetable. I do not eat at night, I haven't in 25 years. This way, I digest my last meal and go to bed with a clean colon. Somewhere in between my small meals, I'll have my recovery drink, which is very filling, and could be considered my fifth meal.

This way of eating is very easy on my digestive system. I eat only what my body can burn and avoid storing calories as fat. As a result, my weight remains steady and I'm never hungry. If you suffer from bloating, constipation, heartburn or other digestive problems, you may consider adding more fiber to your diet in the form of fruits and vegetables, eating smaller meals and avoiding late night eating.

For good nutrition and health—with natural weight loss and maintenance—it is essential to know about, appreciate and prepare the great variety of foods Mother Nature has given us. As we develop our strength and energy through training, we must feed our body the freshest, most nutritious and delicious foods. Our body will always welcome these essential nutrients for maintenance and recovery.

VITAMINS AND MINERALS

Everyone needs vitamins, and athletes especially need more vitamins than non-athletes. In order to perform at peak levels—whether at the gym, the track or throughout your day—we need to provide our body with the appropriate amount of vitamins and minerals. Hardly anyone eats enough food to absorb the nutrients necessary for a body's peak performance and recuperation.

I believe strongly in the importance of adding vitamin supplements to our diets. I take vitamins every day because my diet alone does not always satisfy my necessary nutrient requirements. For example, I've been taking between 5,000 milligrams to 10,000 milligrams of Vitamin C for the last 20 years.

In his book, *How to Live Longer and Feel Better*,[19] Dr. Linus Pauling says that to improve health and prolong life, adults need to take 6 grams (6,000 mgs.) to 18 grams (18,000 mgs.) of vitamin C per day.[20] I began with 2,000 milligrams and have gradually increased that amount over time.

My skin reveals the benefits of my daily intake of Vitamin C every day In spite of my age—70 at this writing—my skin has retained most of its elasticity and resiliency. Vitamin C strengthens the collagen and elastin that supports my skin. Though typical to even middle age, I have avoided developing brown age spots caused by free-radicals. Free-radicals are a by-product of metabolism, but they also are found in toxins, pollution, cigarette smoke and fried foods. Vitamin C is a potent anti-oxidant that neutralizes the damaging effects of free-radicals in the body, thus preventing the formation of brown age spots.

I also heal very fast. Vitamin C aids in wound healing and helps skin rejuvenate. Some doctors recommend Vitamin C supplementation after surgery.

My Vitamin C use shares an example of how such supplementation can be supportive to elastic and resilient skin. However, I am not endorsing this practice but rather

---

[19] Pauling, Linus Ph.D., *How to Live Longer and Feel Better* (Corvallis, OR: Oregon State University Press, 1986)

[20] Ibid, p. 8

encouraging my readers to inform themselves as to the benefits of taking vitamins.

My purpose in this chapter has been to share my personal nutritional practices to help my readers in their quest for greater health, freedom from disease and longevity.

Be a conscious eater. Seek pleasure in selecting the most nutritious foods, cook as if feeding a queen or king and make eating a celebration of your life and health.

ᔕ

CHAPTER SEVEN
Managing Your Stress

*"A spiritual person is one who lives fully in the present moment,
which means living fully in the body. Maharishi inspired me
to see that using meditation as a way to defeat aging was a
legitimate spiritual goal."* [1]

—Deepak Chopra, M.D.

(Deepak Chopra is a world-renowned authority in the field of mind-body healing, a
best-selling author, and the founder of the Chopra Center for Wellbeing.)

S tress is our body's natural reaction to perceived danger and
also a threat to our body's equilibrium—its rate of wear
and tear. Stress accelerates many aspects of the aging process.

Everything in life is stressful by matter of degree. Simply
climbing a step is stressful to the body. Sending our brain the
message to lift our leg creates a tiny amount of cellular activity,
a form of stress. For most people, climbing a step doesn't feel
stressful, certainly not as stressful as tripping down the stairs,
but both events activate parts of the same pathways in the body
and brain.

<hr>

[1] Chopra, Deepak. *Ageless Body, Timeless Mind* (New York: Harmony Books,
1993) p. 167

131

I believe stress is anything we wish were different. For example, when we feel out of sorts, unhappy with our self, our job, our home, our family, perhaps feeling more rejected than accepted, we experience undue stress.

Noted endocrinologist Hans Selye coined the term "stress" more than 70 years ago, when he stated in his book *The Stress of Life*, "No one can live without experiencing some degree of stress all the time. It is false to think that only serious disease or mental or physical injury can cause stress."

He explained that the body, in spite of all the demands placed on it, struggles to maintain its balance. It does so through three stages he called the "general adaptation syndrome."[2]

The first stage is the alarm stage, also known as the fight-or-flight response. We've all felt this, for example, perhaps we've slammed on brakes to avoid hitting a child on a bike that suddenly crossed our path. Our heart pounded, our palms got sweaty, our muscles tensed. We held our breath and stress hormones surged through us—the body's way of providing us with instant energy to handle the emergency.

The second phase, the resistance stage, begins when, having handled the situation, our body expects some recovery and repair. In its determination to keep us healthy, the body perpetually seeks a return to balance. At this phase, our hormonal levels may have returned to normal, but our immune defenses have been challenged and our energy level depleted.

However, if the stressful situation persists, our resistance will be further worn down, and our body will adapt by remaining in a state of arousal. If this persistence of arousal without recovery

---

[2] Selye, Hans, M.D. *The Stress of Life* (New York: McGraw-Hill Book Co., 1984) p. 276

happens repeatedly, health problems will begin to appear.

Consistent hormonal overload can damage both our hearts and our brain. Too much adrenaline can spike blood pressure that can damage blood vessels in both our heart and brain and excess cortisol can damage our cells and muscle tissues. Adrenaline and cortisol are just two of the hormones our body uses in stressful situations. Adrenaline provides a quick boost of energy and activates the fight-or-flight response and cortisol gives us the endurance to stay alert during the crisis.

Hormonal overload can also cause your telomeres to suffer.

Telomeres are the tips at the end of our chromosomes that keep our DNA from unraveling. Each time one of our cells reproduces our telomeres shorten. Excessive stress can damage our telomeres, leaving our DNA unprotected so that it begins to fray. This causes our cells to stop dividing, growing and replenishing our body.

We can influence the size of our telomeres by reducing the effects of stress on our body. We can keep our cells healthy by practicing stress reduction techniques.

It is now widely accepted in the scientific community—by Dr. Walter M. Bortz II, M. D., author of *The Roadmap to 100*, for one—that the length of telomeres marks the age of our cells and our whole organism. Short telomeres indicate older and more exhausted cells. According to Dr. Michael Roizen and Dr. Mehmet Oz, authors of *YOU: Staying Young*, the telomeres of stressed people are almost 50 percent shorter than people who claim they are not stressed. Stressed bodies then are 9 to 17 years older than those who are without stress!

The final and most dangerous stage of the general adaptation syndrome is the exhaustion phase. By now stress has become unrelenting, causing depletion of the body's energy. Such stress overload risks a host of serious illnesses and mishaps like auto accidents. Chronic stress damages the hippocampus section of our brain, impairing memory capabilities and leading to anxiety and depression. Chronic stress also contributes to the accumulation of fat in the abdominal area, also known as "belly fat syndrome," which can lead to heart disease.

Years ago, Sylvia, a client in her mid-50s, had suddenly developed asthma, a disease rare in adults. One afternoon, as we relaxed for a moment after an exercise session, she asked me if I had any idea why she'd gotten sick. "You might want to look at the stress in your life," I said casually. Alarmed, Sylvia jumped out of her chair and burst out: "There's *no* stress in my life!"

But her "perfect life," as she described it, involved driving 90 miles to another town to babysit her grandchildren three times each week. She did not consider long-distance driving three times per week to be stressful, but her body evidently did. Now, at the insistence of her doctor, she had begun my exercise class. Not since the birth of her first grandchild six years before had she taken the time for physical activity, and now only at her doctor's urging.

Like Sylvia, most of us think that only high-level disasters like divorce, job loss, a move or a death in the family are stressful. In fact, in addition to the fairly low-level, but perpetual stress of job and family duties, the accumulation of hovering unfinished details can be equally damaging to our bodies.

COMMON SIGNS OF STRESS

How can we tell if we're stressed out? The most common symptoms are shoulder, neck and back pain. According to Dr. Mehmet Oz and Dr. Michael F. Roizen, authors of *YOU: The Owner's Manual*, about 65 million Americans suffer from back pain, the second most common reason for medical visits. Other common signs of stress are: grinding of the teeth, headaches, insomnia, chronic fatigue, skin rashes, outbursts of emotion, unsteady hands and achy, tight muscles. We're a tense, wired-tight society.

Stress affects us mentally, emotionally and physically. We lose our focus, become forgetful and confused, angry and frustrated. We develop back and shoulder pain. We worry about whether things will ever be peaceful, and if not, how we will cope.

In our despair, we try to console ourselves by flopping on the couch with a pizza or we watch TV. We shop or get lost on the computer. We don't resolve the stress and carry its consequences inside our bodies from one day to the next, hoping to escape a frightening diagnosis.

On the other hand, some stress can be beneficial. Stress can motivate us to do more than we think we can do. This reminds me of the mother who lifted the front end of the car to free her child from potential harm or the pedestrian who raced into oncoming traffic to save a child from being run over. Dr. Selye refers to good stress as "eustress." In limited and manageable doses, stress can actually makes us stronger.

We must, however, know our limits, and be very respectful and attuned to our body's levels of discomfort. This allows us to recognize warning signs of distress—eyelid spasms, shivers throughout the body, floaters dancing in our field of vision or excessive sneezing—and to "dial down" our stress level to prevent ourselves from getting sick.

MY KATRINA LESSON

I learned this lesson back in 2005 after I arrived back home in New Orleans about six weeks after Katrina had hit. As building manager of our 100-year-old Victorian building in the University section of New Orleans, I was eager to begin the reconstruction process. I was responsible for dealing with the insurance company and managing the repairs, which included securing roofers, carpenters who could install sheet-rock and painters.

Having spent much of my evacuation time learning about roofing materials, locating and hiring roofers and communicating with my insurance assessor, I arrived in New Orleans prepared—a good thing since customers outnumbered repairmen a thousand to one.

I knew from neighborhood friends to expect the worst on our building's exterior, but I was not prepared for the extent of damage inside the building. In my second-floor living room, I could see the sky through an eight-foot-square hole in the ceiling and an inch of dust covered everything.

I lived without a roof for two months until the new one was installed. In the meantime, I had to be hyper-vigilant for signs of rain, because the rain poured straight through the hole into my living room. To protect my floors and prevent the whole condo from flooding, I had to cover the floors with anything I could find that could hold or soak water—pots, pans, towels and blankets. I spent many hours emptying pots and pans and wringing wet towels and blankets dry.

Throughout this ordeal I kept thinking that if Katrina had happened to me before I changed my life—when I was physically unfit and handled crisis by retreating and worrying—the experience would have destroyed me. Instead, I replaced my former panic and hopelessness with calm, determined action.

I could not have survived Katrina without meditation, exercise and affirmations. Every day I meditated, prayed for resolution of the countless problems I faced, used affirmations to stay positive and exercised regularly. I knew what elevated levels of dangerous hormones could do to my body and was determined to exercise the tension out. Together, all of these practices saved me. They kept my stress level within manageable limits and prevented me from getting sick.

In the end, Katrina made me stronger and inoculated me against future stresses. I knew then that if I could survive Katrina, I could survive anything! In a way, I'm actually grateful to Katrina because it forced me to do things I didn't think I could do.

STRESS MANAGEMENT TECHNIQUES

Extremely stressful situations are simply part of life. We've all experienced them. The key to surviving such challenges depends upon having and using tools that help us emerge from the situation empowered, instead of demoralized. The following tools allow us to neutralize potentially dangerous effects of stress in a healthy way. We can practice these techniques anywhere, anytime, to maintain our body's equilibrium and remain healthy.

Deep Breathe. When we're stressed, worried or frightened, our "sympathetic" nervous system kicks in and we hold our breath or breathe irregularly. This type of breathing originates from the chest, neck and shoulders. It raises our heart rate and blood pressure and sends a message to the immune system that danger lurks, warning, "Be anxious!"

By contrast, deep breathing—relaxed and slow—also known as diaphragmatic breathing, originates in the abdomen. Deep breathing stimulates the body's "parasympathetic" reaction that calms us down and sends a message to the immune system that "It's okay to relax now."

It's been scientifically proven that deep breathing improves the functioning of the heart, the brain, digestion, the immune system and possibly the effect or action produced by genes. Breathing exercises can lower blood pressure, heart rate and pulse as well as boost immunity.

To practice abdominal breathing, sit or lie down comfortably. Put one hand on your chest and the other on your stomach. Slowly inhale through your nose. As you inhale, feel your stomach expand. Slowly exhale through pursed lips to regulate the release of air. Feel your stomach contract. Rest and repeat. Keep breathing slowly and deeply until you feel relaxed or you have regained your composure.

Meditate. Practicing meditation on a regular basis slows aging at the cellular level and neutralizes the potential damage caused by stress hormones, thus prolonging life. The benefits of meditation far outweigh the time and effort that a few minutes of quiet time takes every day. Our body welcomes these moments of silence that clear the mind and create inner peace while lowering the risk of disease.

I have been meditating for 20 years and strongly recommend it. More than only relieving stress, it clears my mind, improves my memory and eases facial lines. Meditation has allowed me to experience the workings of my mind so I can explore what prompts my thoughts, feelings and actions. Meditation can transform negative behavior patterns that might otherwise keep us from moving forward.

For example, if I feel uncomfortable around someone, I wonder if it's because I'm holding on to something about that person that I need to resolve and release. I meditate and ask myself why I am feeling this way and what unconscious thoughts are driving these distressing feelings? I then pray for guidance.

Once I witness my discomfort and inquire about it in meditation and ask for guidance, an insight usually reveals its wisdom as thought or image. This may bring a shift in perception and ease an otherwise stressful situation, bringing life back into balance.

Not long ago I experienced a very disturbing situation with a neighbor. We needed to paint our building, located only two feet from the property line. I'd asked our next-door neighbor for permission to use her yard so we could paint more easily. Then the painters took longer than she liked and she wanted her yard back. I thought the neighbor was petty and she felt violated. The situation had the potential to turn us into enemies.

But I didn't want to live next door to an enemy. So I sat in meditation and asked for guidance. I felt I wanted to be happy rather than right. Within a few minutes of sitting quietly, I felt a softening of my heart. I knew that I needed to apologize to Sue, regardless of who was right or wrong. I bought a beautiful plant and wrote her a note of apology. To my complete surprise, she also apologized. She even admitted that sometimes "I get pulled in the wrong direction."

Besides helping us to self-regulate our emotions, meditation can also be a potent anti-aging tool.

Through meditation we can nurture the flow of *prana* or life force, and direct it to renew and rebuild our cells. Our cells continually break down and replace themselves. Considering that what we focus on increases, when we focus on the rebuilding process, we remain in a state of constant renewal and regeneration, rather than giving our attention to breaking down and inevitable decay. Awareness is a creative force that can foster health and well-being.

Our skin restores itself once each week, our stomach lining every five days, our liver every six weeks and our skeleton every three months. If we experience our body as a bundle of pulsating and vibrating atoms of energy and information, what we are at a subatomic level, and maintain constant communication with our body, we inspire its renewal and vigor while encouraging our body to retain its youthfulness.

I learned to see and experience my body like this from Dr. Deepak Chopra, author of *Ageless Body, Timeless Mind.* "We can change our biology by what we think and feel," he says, "mind influences every cell in our body." Dr. Chopra explains that even though we think of our bodies as being the same from day to day, the truth is that every part of us is always in flux. Every year, 98 percent of the atoms in our bodies will have been replaced by new ones.

If that is the case, why do we then keep recreating the same body with the same physical conditions? Because we have been culturally conditioned to believe the mind and body are separate and that we are victims of sickness and decay. But we can change that old line of thinking and become aware of the power of our minds and the power of awareness to tap into the flow of intelligence running through our bodies. Up until I learned differently from Dr. Chopra's wisdom, I also believed in the social conditioning that sees the body as a machine instead of a living organism.

"Your cells," says Dr. Chopra, "are constantly processing experience and metabolizing it according to your personal views." We *physically* become our judgments as we internalize them.

If we fear getting old and focus on our wrinkles, slowed metabolism and disappearing energy, our biochemical profile will be negatively altered. Our beliefs will become self-fulfilling prophecies. Our body will suffer and we will grow old quickly.

But, if we exercise every day, eat nutritionally and meditate to relieve stress, we will be more likely to live life with joy and a great deal more energy. Our physical body reflects our biological state and we can be younger than our chronological age.

Let me show you how you can use your power of awareness to help your body stay balanced and renewed. This is a meditation I practice every day, based on the fact that we are, at our most basic subatomic level, beings of vibrating energy and information. It's designed to keep my body constantly rebuilding itself. I invite you to join me in a short version.

Sit with your back supported by a wall or pillow. Close your eyes and take five or six deep, slow breaths. Each time you exhale imagine your stress and confusion leaving your body through your toes. Feel your body slowly letting go of all tension. The more relaxed you become, the lighter your body feels. You feel like you're floating. Allow your body to float out of your room, into wide-open space, over the clouds and ocean waves. The further you float out into the ether, the more relaxed you feel. A sense of freedom and joy overtakes you. Your body no longer feels like solid matter, it's now a pulsating bundle of vibrating energy, absorbing healing energy from the universe, reorganizing and rebuilding itself. Hold that vision for a few minutes and allow your body to become solid matter again, as you slowly return to your room. Breathe again, and slowly open your eyes.

Aging, says Dr. Chopra, is nothing more than deviation from the balanced, stable and self-renewing state that we can create for ourselves daily. When we experience physical changes—a new set of wrinkles, less energy and more stiffness—it is likely we have instigated just that through neglect of our awareness. "There's no biochemistry outside awareness," writes Dr. Chopra. Simply said, what we don't use, we lose.

I first read Dr. Chopra's book, *Ageless Body, Timeless Mind*, almost 20 years ago. I pick it up every now and then and reread some of the passages that at the time expanded my awareness about the aging process. I am reminded once again that since my essence is eternal spirit, fear of aging is totally unnecessary. As spirit, my goal is evolution to a higher level of consciousness.

Over the years meditation has been my counselor, my guide and my inspiration. It's like having a session with the wisest part of me, my higher self. You have that wise part within you too. All you have to do is get in touch with it.

There are many ways to meditate. You can simply sit quietly while breathing deeply and focus on your breath as it moves in and out of your nostrils. Or, another approach suggests focusing on a spot between your brows, which is also known as the "third eye". When you notice thoughts flooding your mind—and you will—just let them pass and return to your point of focus. Repeat. Start with five minutes daily and gradually increase your meditation time, as you feel ready. The more you practice, the more natural it will feel. Eventually you'll begin to feel the tension leaving your body, like air being let out of a balloon.

Perhaps you'll decide to take a beginning meditation class or listen to a meditation tape. A class can give you support and structure, while a tape provides convenience. Choose the approach that works best for you. (See my bibliography for suggested reading on this subject.)

Change your attitude. There's nothing more stressful than moving through life with a negative attitude. Complaining, judging and criticizing are all debilitating habits that leave us drained of energy. Remember, stress does not reside only in what happens to you, but in your *perception* of what happens to you. People "get away" from their problems by going on vacation to a beautiful island somewhere, but the truth is, we carry our problems with us wherever we go—in our minds.

We can choose how we respond to what happens to us. Whenever a stressor agitates you, shift your perception from despair to gratitude. Perhaps there's a lesson in the crisis that will make you stronger and wiser. Life wastes nothing.

Exercise. Since the purpose of the fight-or-flight response is to mobilize us to act, physical activity is the natural way to prevent the negative consequences of stress. Not only does exercise control the emotional and physical feelings of stress, but it also works at the cellular level.

Exercise replaces stress with energy. It dissipates stress through breathing and workings muscles. Make exercise a regular part of your life and your stress will quickly fade.

Express Yourself. Our mental and emotional health requires that we freely express our thoughts, feelings and emotions. When we repress this natural process, we hold enormous tension in the body as anger and frustration. And to compound matters, we beat ourselves up for not speaking up, for not taking a stand.

I spent many years swallowing my anger and despising myself for not speaking up. Even telemarketers intimidated me! One persistent salesman called me nearly every day. Finally, I decided enough was enough. The next time he called, I told him to call me back in a few days so I could build up the courage to say "No!" Then I rehearsed saying "No!" directly into the telephone mouthpiece. When the telemarketer called back, I was ready with "No, I'm not interested!"—my voice clear and firm. Elated, I couldn't wait to do it again. Each time, it became easier and easier to say what I meant—not just with telemarketers but with the important people in my life.

These techniques represent only a few of the many that you can practice daily to reduce the stress in your life. Remember that the effects of stress are cumulative, leading to a broad array of health problems. You cannot run away from stress, but you can control the damage it causes by how you meet it when it comes. You can build and strengthen your resiliency to stress, and that, too, is also cumulative. Keep practicing these tools and watch your energy rise, your peacefulness deepen and your overall health and sense of well-being improve.

୯ର

CHAPTER EIGHT
The Forever Fit and Fabulous Generation

"The mind's first step to self-awareness must be through the body."

—Dr. George Sheehan (1918-1993)

(Dr. George Sheehan was an avid runner, author and philosopher. At age 50, Dr. Sheehan ran a 4:47 mile—the world's first sub-five-minute time—by a 50-year-old. He lectured widely on health and fitness.)

The ten people in this Chapter, all devoted clients, are also dedicated athletes. Ranging in ages from 25 to 81, they exemplify health and fitness. They have been working out from 14 months to 20 years. Some of them work-out twice each week, some three and five times per week.

Neither illness nor injury derail their commitment to good health. They experience these as only temporary setbacks and know that getting back on schedule with their exercise routine is the best medicine.

They all share common goals: staying healthy, generating optimum energy for doing all they want to and keeping a youthful glow throughout their lives.

When I ask them what drives their dedication, they all simply say: because it makes me feel and look better, and I have accomplished more than I ever expected.

I feel privileged to have been invited into their lives to share my fitness philosophy. It gives me continued satisfaction to witness their progress. To hear the words: "I feel better" makes my day.

As you, dear readers, make your gains with my Vibrant Health Workout program, I hope to hear from you. May you too unleash your inner athlete and become stronger, healthier and happier than you have ever been.

EMMA, Age 25

(Personal assistant to media personality)

I've been weight training for four years.

I began training during my senior year in college as a way to get healthy and lose weight. I started doing a mixture of cardio-aerobic exercise and lifting free weights and found that I immediately noticed a difference in my energy and stress level. Gradually, I also began to lose weight and re-shape my body but the change that I most noticed and enjoyed has been a new sense of awareness and control of my body. Particularly as I advanced to lifting heavier weights and performing more challenging exercises, I felt more capable of handling everyday physical challenges and therefore more

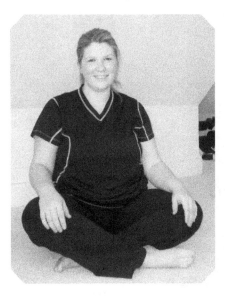

freedom to participate in types of activities that I may not have previously been drawn to.

Over the past four years that I have been training, I have graduated from college and shifted my life towards a demanding professional career. Through this time period and many life changes, my consistency with exercise has varied but I know that when I am able to follow a regular training program, I am far more mentally and physically prepared to face future challenges.

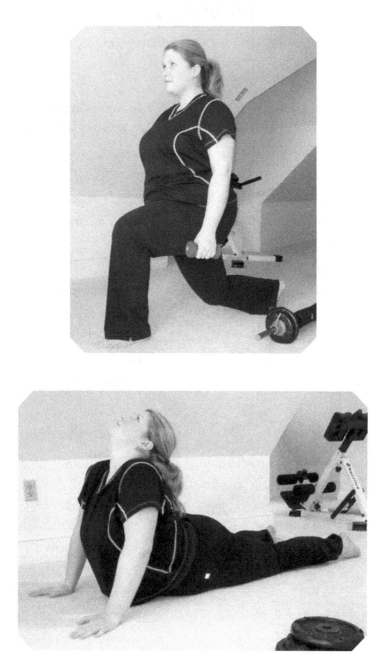

JACKIE, age 76

(Real estate lawyer)

Why workout? So I can still touch my toes when I am 100 years old!

On the next page, I am doing my favorite exercise, chest flyes, with 25 pounds and my favorite stretch, the split!

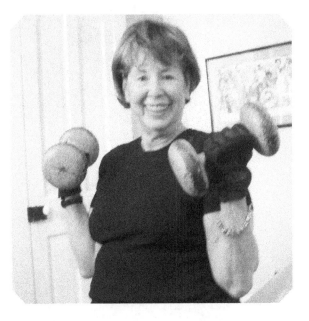

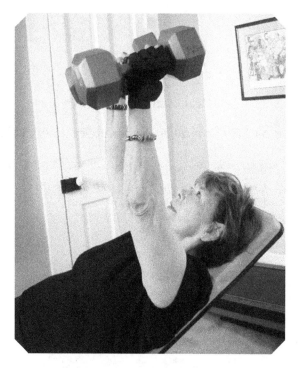

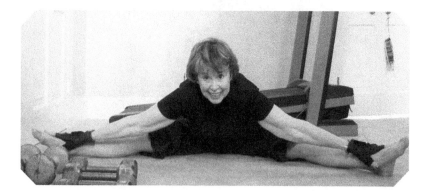

SANDY, age 62

(Horseback riding and jumping enthusiast)

I believe that the most powerful method of enhancing mental and physical well-being is the weight training that I have been enjoying for the last 12 years. It has allowed me to take up the challenging sport of horseback riding and jumping that I embarked upon five years ago.

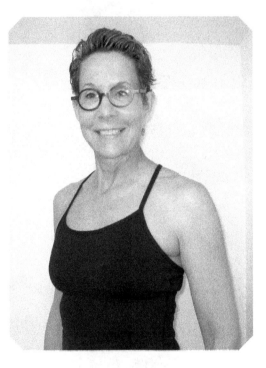

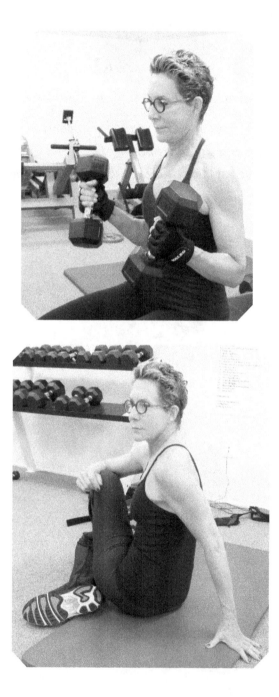

BRUCE, age 63
(Cardiologist)

Weight training has been my mistress and psychologist for the last ten years. She's challenging, but always makes me look and feel better.

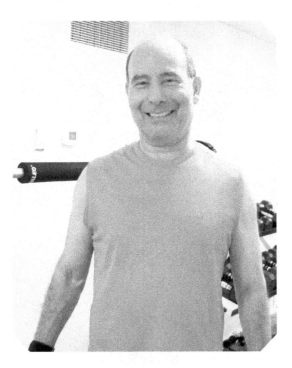

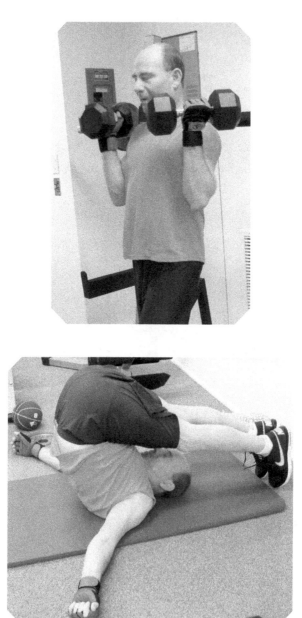

RODNEY, Age 81
(Hotelier)

I've been working out since I was 60. Some would say it was a late start, but it was a wonderful beginning. I have more strength, stamina and energy now than when I began 20 years ago. I look forward to every workout and never miss one, except when I'm traveling. Consistency is the key.

My stretch routine includes lots of lower-back stretching exercises. On the next page I am strengthening my deltoids with 30-pound dumbbells.

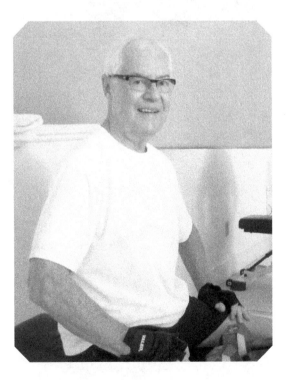

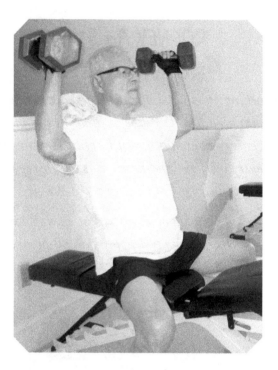

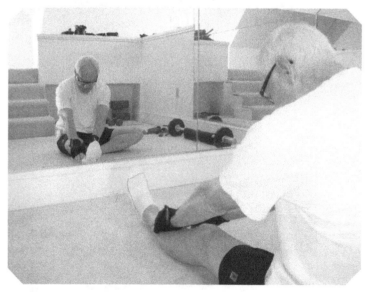

TINA, age 62

(Lawyer)

I have been training for 10 months. Before I began I had a series of non-life-threatening but debilitating illnesses, but now I have more strength, stamina and energy than I thought I would ever have again. The results of working out gratify me and working with weights has become a pleasure. I love getting acquainted with my individual muscles and feeling them work, stretch and grow.

On the next page I'm doing the biceps curl with 15 pounds and it's a challenge, but I love it!

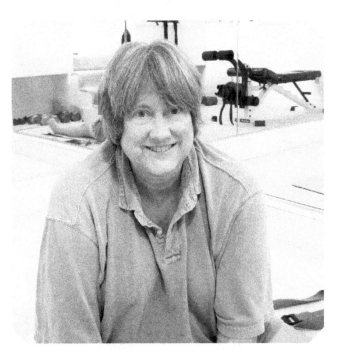

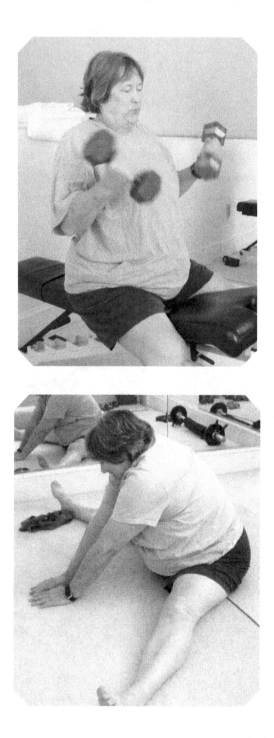

CHERYL, age 55

(Lawyer)

I have been working out with Emelina for six months. I have not only increased my strength and vitality but my quality of life has also been greatly enhanced.

During this time, I have also lost 25 pounds and my joints no longer ache. Keeping up with my workouts has made me realize I have the inner discipline and determination to get healthier and stronger as I age, and that life can be deluxe, no matter how old I live to be.

On the next page I am doing chest presses with 25-pound dumbbells!

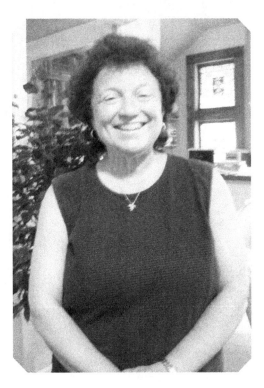

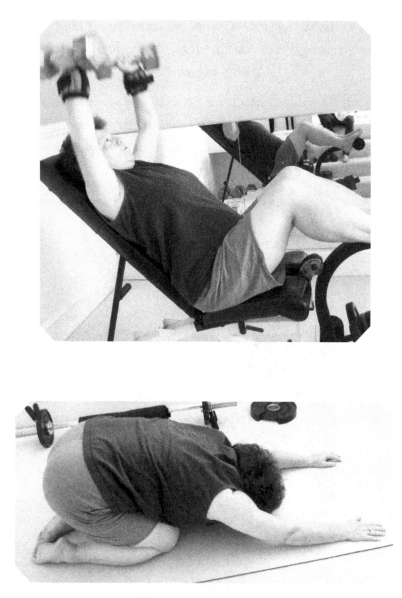

LARRY, Age 65

(Eye Surgeon)

After working out for 12 years I am 20 pounds lighter and five years younger! I've struggled with tight hamstrings that affect my lower back, so on the next page I am doing hamstring stretches for flexibility and dead lifts to strengthen my lower back.

Stretching on a regular basis has actually increased my strength due to a greater range of motion. My muscles can now generate greater force and that means more power throughout all of my movements.

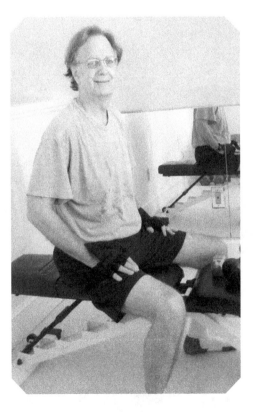

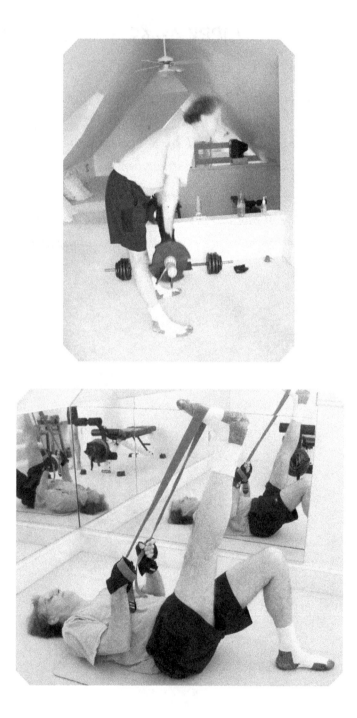

PEGGY, Age 62

(Psychotherapist)

I started weight training 12 years ago just before my 50th birthday. Weight training with Emelina took me into an amazing world that offered strength I could not have predicted. I have continued to "test" the higher weights and surprise myself over and over. My posture has improved along with my conscious breathing, both during the workout and throughout my day. The echo of Emelina's words, "Yes I can!" and "Strength and Energy!" have become embedded in my psyche. They motivate me to keep going in other settings like both of the 150-mile MS Tour for Cure Bike Rides I have done.

On the next page I am doing triceps extensions with 20 pounds and doing bridge, my favorite stretch.

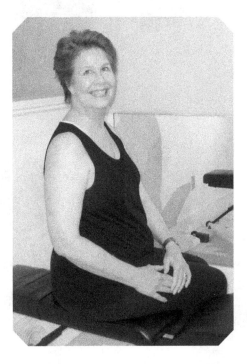

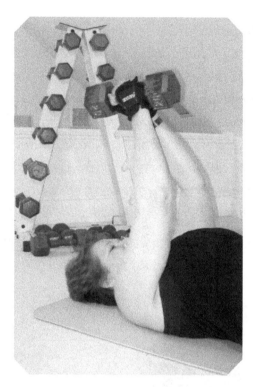

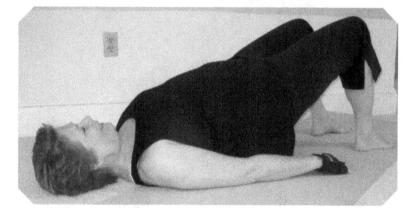

CAROLYN, *age 60*

(Licensed clinical social worker, Ph.D.)

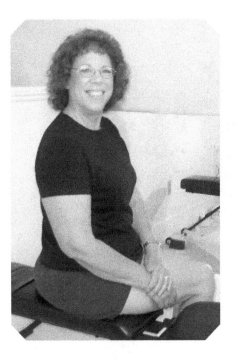

After recovering from Achilles tendon surgery at age 57, I was weak, out of shape and overweight. During a safari trip in South Africa, a colleague invited me to join in a "mild" hike to see ancient Indian rock paintings. Fear told me I wasn't in shape to do this hike. But my sense of adventure, encouragement from my friend and reassurance that the hike was "mild" won me over. The rock paintings were amazing! But after seven hours of hiking a "not-so-mild" hike, hobbling down the hill with support on both sides, knees shaking and exhausted, I said to myself, "Wow, are you out of shape!" followed by, "But you still did it. Imagine how your body would perform if you actually got into shape!"

Now, after two years of weight lifting, stretching, losing 45 pounds and hiking to the top of a Himalayan mountain, I can say, "Weight lifting didn't save my life, but it definitely saved my Active Life."

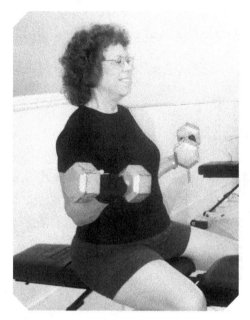

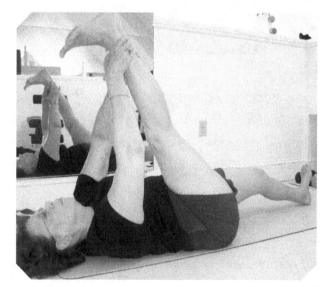

CHAPTER NINE
For the Love of It

"If you could only love enough, you could be the most powerful person in the world."

—Emmett Fox (1886-1951)

(Dr. Emmett Fox is one of the most influential spiritual leaders of the 20th Century.)

I never dreamed when I started training 25 years ago that, at 70, I'd be stronger and look better than ever before.

I had no expectations when I started. I trained because I knew it was necessary for my good health and well-being. I never looked further than the present moment and trained for the love of it.

In addition to letting go of expectations, I told myself that since I had no place to go but where I was, then why not invest my time in rebuilding my life—while lifting weights?

To find myself today feeling and looking better than ten years ago when I turned 60, is a fantastic gift. My strength does not surprise me, but the youthful appearance is a *lagniappe* (a little something extra).

Throughout the years scientific research has given us more and more reason to pick up weights and build muscle. They convinced me from the get go and I've been happy to oblige ever since.

Twenty-five years sounds like a long time, but lived fully present day by day, it feels as short as one day.

Imagine if I had not listened to my inner voice. Today I may not be here. And if I'd made it, I'd be an unhealthy mess.

Listen to your inner voice when it speaks to you. It's the voice of wisdom. Don't wait another day. Time doesn't stop and aging waits for no one. You can change your body. You can become stronger, healthier and more youthful than yesterday. Five, then ten years from now you will look back grateful for following your voice of wisdom.

SLOWING THE AGING PROCESS

The pictures on the facing page were taken 22 years apart. In the picture on the left, I am 47. In the picture on the right I am 70.

I am stronger at 70, than I was at 47. Today I can do chest presses with 35-pound dumbbells (back then I was lifting 30 pounds), and I can squat with a 90-, 95- and 100-pound barbell. I do 40-50 reps. I believe in exertion. After a strenuous workout, I feel relaxed, energized, content and proud of my accomplishment. Training enables me to move effortlessly, to have a pain-free body and prevent illness (I haven't been sick in bed in 20 years).

☙

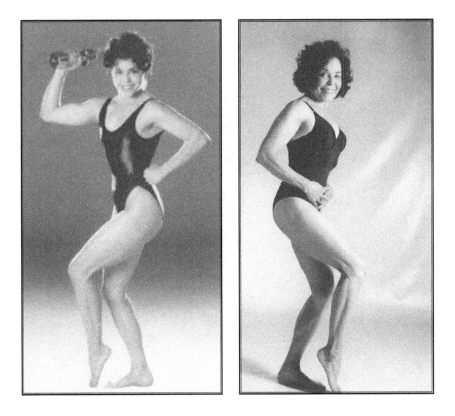

CHAPTER TEN
Your Body, Your Gateway to Spirit

"There is more wisdom in your body than in your deepest philosophy".

—Friedrich Nietzsche (1844-1900)

(Nineteenth century German philosopher and poet)

Exercise conditions the body, toughens the mind and nourishes the spirit.

When we begin to train our body, we begin a process that can eventually lead to our most powerful self. Once mind, body and spirit are one, we can take on what before seemed impossible.

Each time we challenge our self to lift more weight or learn an advanced exercise we are awakening parts of us—determination, discipline, power, commitment—that may have lain dormant for many years. We build mental strength in the process and this leads to resiliency, our insurance against life's challenges.

I remember vividly the first time I walked into a gym. It took all the courage I could muster to walk in the front door. I was so self-conscious that I wanted to hide from prying eyes. I thought all eyes were on me. I didn't want anyone to see how awful I looked. I was ashamed of my body. My chest was sunken and my back bowed. I felt old. My energy was so depleted; I had barely made it out of bed that morning.

A "for women only" sign caught my eye. I felt instant relief: an isolated area set aside for women only. The area reserved for women was both isolated and empty. I walked up three narrow steps, opened my weight-training book, picked up a set of weights and began to lift. I sought refuge in my regular visits to the gym.

With each lift of the weight and increase in load, my confidence grew. I gradually began to feel better about myself. No longer obsessed with how I looked or my wish to be invisible, I began to notice my newly developing muscles and overall muscular strength. My feet no longer shuffled across the floor, I lifted my legs with quad strength.

One day I ventured out of my little spot to explore other areas of the gym. I met other exercisers and began to smile and say hello. When I finally let my guard down, I realized no one was looking at me with critical eyes; they couldn't have cared less what I looked like. For me, that was a phenomenal realization. I had projected my own negative self-assessment on to others.

In just a few months I had gained strength of mind, body and spirit. I felt hopeful for my future and began to trust that the universe would provide, as long as I energetically pushed forward and continued to challenge myself.

Weight training became my life coach. You too can embrace this new approach to total well-being by developing more muscle strength, learning new exercise moves and perhaps awakening dormant spiritual qualities. You too can be the recipient of such a magnificent gift.

I've seen it happen countless times. Newcomers who spend time getting to know their bodies and testing their strength surprise themselves. They realize they're stronger than their limited expectations. Grateful for and in awe of what their bodies can do, they leave their first experience feeling better than when they started. I can always expect to hear the usual "I feel so much better already."

It doesn't take very long before the newcomer confidence soars. Within a few months strength levels usually double. For example, a client may tell me that she can now lift potted plants where before she could not. Or, she can now move a piece of furniture without asking for help. Apparent pride in new accomplishments fuels satisfaction and excitement and generates commitment to continue.

The more we challenge ourselves physically, I believe, the greater the spiritual benefit.

Many years ago I read an inspiring story about the long-distance swimmer Diana Nyad. In 1979, Diana swam from the island of Bimini to Florida—more than 100 miles—and set a world record. A few years earlier she had set another record. She circled Manhattan in a record time of 7 hours, 57 seconds. When asked why? Why train so hard to do that? She replied, "Because it builds character."

I want that, I remember thinking at the time. I want *character*.

The word "character" struck a chord within me. In my old life I had been weak, afraid to speak up for myself, dependent on others for my sense of worth and quick to please. Even though I had become a bit more assertive and confident since I had begun training, I still wrestled with my timidity. I was still holding back my power. I wanted a strong mind, body and spirit. I wanted the fearless mentality of a yogi. The yogi stands before the world unafraid and securely able to influence his destiny.

Diana retired for a few years, but when her 60th birthday came she felt the need to motivate herself again. She still imagined a Cuba swim, a challenge that had eluded her in the past. "I wanted to feel unwavering commitment again," she said, "I wanted to feel like my best days were not behind me." After a year of training, she doesn't feel old anymore but stronger than she did at 20.[1]

Note: As of August 9, 2011, Diana was forced to abandon her 103-mile Florida to Cuba swim. After swimming for nearly 29 hours, at about the halfway point, she could no longer endure her shoulder pain and asthma attacks, in the midst of threatening ocean swells, and reluctantly ended her quest. Her effort would have been the first such swim without a shark cage. To have given it her all, and stayed in the ocean for that length of time, still makes her a hero in my eyes, even though she didn't complete her intended goal.

Between the times the word "character" jolted me into awareness and Katrina put me to the test, I spent many years honing the very traits I knew that I needed to own my place in the world. I reflected on my words and actions every day and examined my reactions to people and events. When not satisfied with the outcome of a particular situation, I vowed to change. I read motivational books voraciously and applied what resonated with me.

After the worst natural disaster in our country's history, I returned to New Orleans ready to prove to myself that I was up

---

[1] http://www.aolnews.com/2010/08/29/at-61-diana-nyad-is-ready-to-swim-from-cuba-to-florida/

to the task. A single, 65-year-old female, I returned to an empty building in an almost vacant neighborhood ready to do the work I had to do. The city's water was undrinkable and the few grocery stores open carried only canned goods. With no doubt, I believed that I could restore the integrity of our beautiful building and take care of myself in the process.

My trajectory in the gym became a metaphor for my evolution in the real world.

Can you identify with either Diana's story or mine? Did you dream once of accomplishing a feat but had to abandon it? What if you began to train your body, developed muscular strength, stamina and resiliency and realized your dream this time around?

To be fit is to be psychologically strong when life knocks us down. We get back up while remaining present and positive, believing that the challenge brings opportunity. Strength of mind, body and spirit is our insurance against all odds.

Our body is the vessel and the vehicle through which we experience our deepest self: our personal power, our courage, our wisdom, our joy, our dreams and our desires.

I challenge and encourage you to begin a workout program, get to know your body and love your body as you would your best friend. See yourself and the world through the eyes of your infinite, highest self. Your life is a miracle, a gift to the world. Honor the sacredness of your existence by honoring your body. Become your own hero by unleashing your innate power. You can be the conqueror of your own life. You have the power to chart its course. It all begins with the wisdom of your body and the great love for who you are.

I love myself; therefore I take care of my body, mind and spirit because everything in my life stems from how I feel about myself.

ɕᴔ

CHAPTER ELEVEN
A New Beginning

"Appreciation of the gift of a body is the first step toward unlocking the spiritual energy available to assist you in your life journey." [1]

—Joyce Whitely Hawkes, Ph.D.

(Internationally renowned biologist and practitioner of traditional Eastern healing methods)

Here we are, at the end of our journey together. I've enjoyed sharing both my struggles and my triumphs with you. I hope my stories have inspired you, as I was once moved and motivated to change by learning how others' triumphed over losses far greater than mine.

For 25 years I've felt grateful and been humbled to inspire and support change in others' lives. Just this morning, Theresa, age 65, a client with only five sessions under her belt, turned to me as we wrapped things up and said, "You have no idea what this

---

[1] Hawkes, Joyce Whitely, Ph.D., *Cell-Level Healing* (New York: Attria Books, 2006) p. xv

workout has done for my confidence. It's not about the weight, heck, I'm only lifting five pounds," she said as she raised one of her dumbbells. "It's about how I feel inside. It's about a new beginning, one where I take charge of my body and my life."

That sentiment describes my wish for you: a new beginning, where you take charge of your body and your life. What else in the world offers anyone such a great reward for such a small investment (one hour a day) in such a short amount of time?

In my introduction I shared that I offered you radical ideas that, when followed, could slow, and in many cases, reverse the decay you may have already experienced. Radical aging, or biologically erasing half your age by how you live your life, is not only a possibility; it's the inevitable consequence of putting your health first on your daily schedule.

You may be wondering how, with your busy life, you will find time for one hour or even half an hour of exercise each day. You can find that hour by reducing or dropping from your daily schedule, activities that are not as important for your health and well-being. For example, forgo TV, computer games (one of my clients divulged when asked, that she spent two to three hours every night playing computer games), late-night office work (your longevity will benefit more from fitness than the stress of overwork) and so on.

Once you have found your daily hour, break it down something like this: five-minute warm-up, 20-minute cardio, 20-minute weights, 10-minute stretching and 5-minute meditation.

Instead of breaking your fitness components (weights, cardio, stretching and meditation) throughout your week and performing them in isolation, combine them into a comprehensive program, and you will make greater gains. Synergistically, mind (meditation), body (exercise) and spirit (self-esteem) will coalesce into a greater whole.

Now decide how many times per week you'll work out: two, three or four. Write it down on your weekly schedule. You might begin with two workouts per week and once you begin to feel stronger and ready for more, make it three. This is how I've trained for 25 years, except today I work out every day (alternating muscle groups). No part of my body or psyche is left behind on any given day.

Somewhere within your week I would recommend reading inspiring literature, particularly motivational books that have the power to take you to the next level of empowerment. You may discover that by changing a negative mental pattern, you can let go of a destructive habit. A steady diet of inspiration and motivation is essential for change to become permanent. And you want for these changes to become who you are. My bibliography offers some amazing choices. Feeding your mind is as important as feeding your body.

If you're not already a vegetarian, begin to experiment with vegetarian dishes and incorporate two or three of these in your diet on a weekly basis. Keep an open mind and allow your taste buds to retrain themselves to new flavors that will benefit your health and energy levels. Slowly begin to distance yourself from alcohol, sugar, salt and fat. Eat pure food. Cleansed is the new order in your life—a clean system for a new beginning.

Nurturing your mind, body and spirit on a daily basis will connect you to your inner power source. Your confidence will increase, your movements will become more fluid, your posture will improve, you'll express your needs more naturally and appreciation and love of self will follow. And everything you've dreamed of will now become a possibility.

രൂ

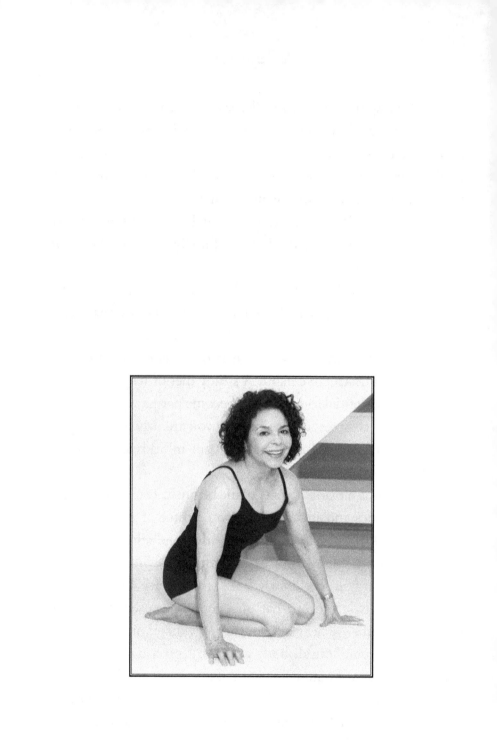

Please Join Me

BECOME A MEMBER OF MY *FOREVER FIT AND FABULOUS* GENERATION—TOGETHER, LET'S CHANGE THE WORLD!

I invite you to join me in turning the *Forever Fit and Fabulous* Generation into a grassroots movement to promote aging with health and vigor. By spreading the word about the benefits of healthy living, especially lifting weights, we can save millions of people from unnecessary suffering.

Imagine a world of healthy, vigorous centenarians enjoying life and having fun, contributing to the betterment of the world instead of sitting in nursing homes deteriorating day by day.

I want to hear from you. Let me know how you're doing. Ask questions. Or simply let me know you're doing fabulously, feeling and looking better by the day.

Let's stay in touch through my website: **fitfabat70.com** and **emelina.com**. I will be posting frequent blogs and creating new products. In the works are a Vibrant Health Workout DVD, a Forever Fit and Fabulous Journal and a companion cookbook. I want to provide you with as many tools as possible to make your journey towards greater health and well being more fun and enjoyable.

Thanks for being my friend. We're all in this together. Let's make this a better world!

℘

Bibliography

Aurobindo, Sri. *The Life Divine*. Twin Lakes: Lotus Press, 1990.

Berg, Yehuda. *The Power of Kabbalah*. Los Angeles: The Kabbakah Center, 2004.

Bloodworth, Venice. *Key To Yourself*. Marina del Rey: DeVorss & Co, 1952.

Bosnak, Robert. *A Little Course in Dreams*. Boston: Shambala Publications, Inc. 1986.

Bradshaw, John. *The Family: A Revolutionary Way of Self-Discovery*. Deerfield Beach: Health Communications, 1988.

Branden, Nathaniel. *Six Pillars of Self-Esteem: The Definitive Work on Self-Esteem by the Leading Pioneer in the Field*. New York: Bantam, 1994.

Bly, Robert. *A Little Book on the Human Shadow*. New York: HarperCollins Publishers, 1988.

Chrystyn, Julie. *The Secret to Life Transformation: How To Claim Your Destiny Now!* Beverly Hills: Dove Books Inc., 2009.

Crowley, Chris and Lodge, Henry S. *Younger Next Year for Women: Turn Back Your Biological Clock*. New York: Workman Publishing, 2005.

De Becker, Gavin. *The Gift of Fear, Survival Signals that Protect Us from Violence.* USA: Little, Brown & Company Limited, 1997.

Dychtwald, Ken. *Bodymind.* New York: Jeremy P. Tarcher/ Putman, 1950.

Emoto, Masaru. *The Hidden Messages in Water.* Hillsboro: Beyond Words Publishing Inc., 2004.

Forward, Susan. *Emotional Blackmail: When the People in Your Life Use Fear, Obligation and Guilt to Manipulate You.* New York: HarperCollins Publishers, 1997.

Foundation for Inner Peace. *A Course in Miracles.* Glen Ellen: Foundation for Inner Peace, 1975.

Fuhrman, Joel. *Eat to Live.* New York: Little, Brown & Company, 2003.

Gould, Roger. *Shrink Yourself: Break Free from Emotional Eating Forever! (The Therapist's Guide to Losing Weight).* Hoboken: John Wiley & Sons Inc., 2007.

Hawkins, David R. *Transcending the Levels of Consciousness: The Stairway to Enlightenment.* W. Sedona: Veritas Publishing, 2006.

Jung, Carl, G. *Memories, Dreams, Reflections.* New York: Vintage Books, 1989.

Mahoney, Maria F. *The Meaning in Dreams and Dreaming.* Secaucus: The Citadel Press, 1966.

McDougall, Christopher. *Born to Run.* New York: Alfred A. Knopf, 2009.

Miller, Alice. *The Body Never Lies: The Lingering Effects of Hurtful Parenting.* New York: W. W. Norton & Co., 2006.

Miller, Alice. *The Drama of the Gifted Child.* New York: Basic Books, 1997.

Pert, Candace. *Molecules of Emotion: Why You Feel the Way You Feel.* New York: Scribner, 1997.

Pittman, Frank. *Grow Up! How Taking Responsibility Can Make You a Happy Adult.* New York: Golden Books, 1998.

Rama, Swami. *Living with the Himalayan Masters.* Honesdale: The Himalayan Institue Press, 2001.

Ratey, John J., with Eric Hagerman. *Spark: The Revolutionary New Science of Exercise and the Brain.* New York: Little, Brown & Company, 2008.

Robbins, Anthony. *Unlimited Power.* New York: Fawcett Columbine, 1986.

Satir, Virginia. *The New People Making.* Mountain View: Science and Behavior Books, Inc., 1988.

Walford, Roy L. and Walford, Lisa. *The Anti-Aging Plan.* New York: Marlowe & Company, 1994.

Whitely Hawkes, Joyce. *Cell-Level Healing: The Bridge from Soul to Cell.* New York: Atria Books, 2006.

Yogananda, Paramahansa. *Autobiography of a Yogi.* Los Angeles: Self-Realization Fellowship, 1974.

Zimbardo, Philip G. *Shyness: What It Is, What To Do About It.* New York: Addison-Wesley Publishing Company, Inc., 1989.

Zukav, Gary. *The Seat of The Soul.* New York: Simon & Schuster 1989.

જી

Index

❧

ABOUT THE AUTHOR

Emelina Edwards, a Fitness Lifestyle Coach for 25 years, embodies the message she delivers—the key to optimum health and timeless aging is a fitness lifestyle, a message shared across media in both Spanish and English, and now in her long-awaited book, *Forever Fit and Fabulous—Even at 70 and Beyond*. Emelina, now 70 herself, is living proof of her prescription for timeless aging.

CPSIA information can be obtained
at www.ICGtesting.com
Printed in the USA
LVHW041052180123
737309LV00004B/362

9 780615 581262